Every Woman's Guide to

HEALTHY, GLOWING SKIN

Every Woman's Guide to

HEALTHY, GLOWING SKIN

Simple Steps to Beautiful Skin at Any Age

LEAH ROTH

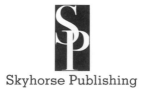

Skyhorse Publishing

Skyhorse Publishing books may be purchased in bulk at special discounts for sales promotion, corporate gifts, fund-raising, or educational purposes. Special editions can also be created to specifications. For details, contact the Special Sales Department, Skyhorse Publishing, 307 West 36th Street, 11th Floor, New York, NY 10018 or info@skyhorsepublishing.com.

Skyhorse® and Skyhorse Publishing® are registered trademarks of Skyhorse Publishing, Inc.®, a Delaware corporation.

Visit our website at www.skyhorsepublishing.com.

10 9 8 7 6 5 4 3 2 1

Library of Congress Cataloging-in-Publication Data

Names: Roth, Leah, author.
Title: Every woman's guide to healthy, glowing skin: simple steps to
    beautiful skin at any age / Leah Roth.
Description: New York, NY: Skyhorse Publishing, [2019]
Identifiers: LCCN 2019001829 | ISBN 9781510742475 (hardback)
Subjects: LCSH: Skin—Care and hygiene—Popular works. | Self-care,
    Health—Popular works. | Beauty, Personal. | BISAC: SELF-HELP / General. |
    HEALTH & FITNESS / Health Care Issues. | SELF-HELP / Aging.
Classification: LCC RL87 .R68 2019 | DDC 646.7/26—dc23 LC record available at
https://lccn.loc.gov/2019001829

Cover design by Mona Lin
Cover illustration by Getty Images

Print ISBN: 978-1-5107-4247-5
Ebook ISBN: 978-1-5107-4252-9

Printed in China

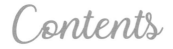

Contents

Introduction

If someone had told me ten years ago (or even one year ago) that I was going to have my first book published at twenty-five years old, I would have laughed . . . and then probably gotten a big ego about it because I would have thought, *I made it big*! The truth is I have not "made it big." I'm just a regular person who was granted a wonderful opportunity. At this very moment I have forty-seven Twitter followers (hint: help a girl out).

I started attending NYU's Gallatin School of Individualized Studies in the fall of 2012 with the intention of majoring in "fashion journalism." I wanted to fulfill my dream of becoming a writer at *Vogue*—their "Five Days, Five Looks, One Girl" segment, which profiled their "cool girl" employees, was my version of crack. Throughout my nearly four years at college, I took several fashion and writing courses. I also interned at *CR Fashion Book*, KCD Worldwide, *Fashionista*, and a few other really cool places.

My specified niche soon expanded, though, as I realized that I was passionate about other things besides high-fashion magazines run by Anna Wintour. I fell in love with the growing movement toward sustainability. I became fascinated by the business side of the industry: supply chain, technology, manufacturing. More important, I, like many other women, grew infatuated with the beauty industry.

Before social media, beauty wasn't so much an obsession as it was a necessity for maintenance and upholding society's unrealistic standards—I actually wrote a very extensive thesis on this premise for my graduation colloquium. Over the past few years, we've seen it unfold into something much bigger. Something few of us could have imagined. Blogs like *Into the Gloss* (yes, *Into the Gloss* used to just be a blog) opened my eyes to the world of cult skincare products, expensive laser treatments, cheap home remedies, and much more. Around this same time, niche beauty brands were popping up everywhere, girls were promoting them on Instagram, and cult branding was (and still is) in full force. Essentially, beauty became so much more than a product; it became a lifestyle. With this transition came a movement toward inclusivity. Beauty started becoming (and is still slowly becoming) a safe space for people of all races, religions, genders, ages, sizes, etc. Beauty doesn't (and shouldn't) discriminate.

After college I worked full-time as a fashion copywriter for two years. When I wasn't struggling to figure out another unique way to upsell $5,000 of polyester (or roasting my coworkers in our group chat), I was reading those same blogs and websites. I had convinced myself over the years that I had lost interest in the world of fashion and beauty, but the truth is, I kept coming back to it. To this day, I still spend an embarrassing amount of time on YouTube watching GRWM videos and makeup tutorials—I mean, really, an excessive amount of time. It's just so fascinating and relaxing. The real world is overwhelming, but the world of beauty provides an escape.

I know I am not alone in my obsession. I wrote this book because I know that there are other people that stay up until 2:00 a.m. on a Sunday night watching smoky eye tutorials instead of preparing for their presentation the next day. I know that there are people who have tried rubbing coconut oil on their face—despite the fact that they knew it would break them out—because everyone else was trying it. I know that there are people who hate on cult skincare brands only to secretly go out and buy their latest product the day it launches. I've learned that it's okay to feel conflicted. Society's relationship with beauty, feminism, and self-care is complicated, so it's only natural for you to question your relationship with the industry as a whole. But caring about "more important" things doesn't mean you can't also care about your skin.

I also wrote this book because I thought there was an untapped space in the market. I know I just mentioned that there's an influx of beauty information, so you may ask, "Why write a book about it?" The answer is: skincare blogs, articles, and social media posts are everywhere online, but it's a lot harder to find something tangible; an informative book that's polished yet feminine. It'll make a great gift for Mother's Day, your best friend's birthday, or your boss who's addicted to facials. Plus, you don't need a WiFi connection—pretty neat, huh? You also don't have to worry about those pesky video ads popping up that you can never figure out how to close out of. For some reason Cialis thinks I'm their target consumer.

At this point in my life, I'm beginning to focus more on writing and comedy—so I hope some of that is reflected in the writing (cue the callback to my Cialis joke two seconds ago). Beauty doesn't have to be taken so seriously. You can want to try the latest face oil trend but still know that you're partially just a victim of good marketing and cute packaging. It's like those astrology meme accounts. Sure, zodiac signs are fun, but they're self-aware about how ridiculous they can be. Do I actually base my life decisions around astrology? No. Am I kidding when I tell people that I'm insecure in romantic relationships because I'm a Taurus? Only a little.

This book covers all of the skincare questions you had but are too embarrassed to ask, can't find a concrete answer to, or didn't even know you had. Chapter 1 is all about the essentials of the everyday face, while chapter 2 delves into treatments for special occasions, and chapter 3 differentiates nighttime versus daytime products. We also discuss skincare for the body, SPF (you're going to get really sick of those three letters), how to read a label, and some classics. While each chapter is distinctly its own, some parts may feel slightly repetitive . . . so feel free to read out of order if that's what floats your boat. Whether you're a beginner or skincare expert, I hope (and think) you'll learn something new from this book. I know I did! That might not be the best for an author to say, but if I hadn't researched anything this wouldn't be a very thorough book, now would it?

If nothing else, I fought really hard to make sure this book looks great on your coffee table—right next to that Le Labo candle your favorite influencer recommended and that Malcolm Gladwell book you read to impress random strangers.

CHAPTER 1

Everyday Face

*L*et's be honest, the world of skincare can be a bit overwhelming. In a market that's overflowing with options, it can be hard to know where to start. Gone are the days when you would walk into your local drugstore and pick up a bar of soap and some sunblock and be on your way. Every time you step into a Sephora or skim through your favorite beauty blog, there's a new product, treatment, or routine that you're convinced you *need* to try. This can lead to a lot of unanswered questions for even the savviest of skincare connoisseurs. Questions like: *What type of cleanser should I be using? Do I need a cleanser at all? Is toner applied before or after moisturizer? Should my morning routine be different from my evening routine?* That's why we've created a guide to help you navigate the basics. Think of this as your everyday face.

Soap vs. Cleanser

A couple of years ago, I told a friend who works in the beauty industry that I only wash my face with soap in the morning, and she looked at me as if I had told her that I had never washed my face in my life. Little did I know that there is a major difference between soap and cleanser. Generally speaking, regular soap contains harsh surfactant ingredients that strip your skin of its natural moisture while cleansers contain synthetic surfactant ingredients, which are milder than regular soap, and can help keep skin healthy and moisturized. In case you don't know, surfactants are chemical compounds that lubricate substances with incompatible molecule properties (like water and oil). Cleansers are also more effective than soap at removing makeup and dirt.

From a scientific standpoint, soap has a general pH level of between nine and ten (the skin is somewhere between four and six), which can make your skin feel clean, but it's often too harsh and irritating. It strips the natural oils from your face, making the pH level too alkaline—this is when your skin often becomes too dry, flaky, or inflamed (ouch). As a result, the sebaceous glands overcompensate and produce too much oil, often resulting in clogged pores and breakouts. Eventually, this can also lead to premature fine lines and wrinkles. Cleansers are at a much lower pH than soap and are gentler on the skin.

Now that we've differentiated between soap and cleanser, you should probably know that there are different types of cleansers as well:

- *Gel cleansers* have—wait for it—a gel-like consistency and provide a deep cleaning without stripping your skin of its natural oils, making it ideal for oily and combination skin. I would guess that if you already own a cleanser, it's probably a gel kind.
- *Cream (or milk) cleaners* are usually thick and contain moisturizing ingredients like botanical oils. They tend to be much gentler and are therefore ideal for dry and sensitive skin.
- *Foam cleansers* start out as a liquid or a gel and turn into a frothy lather. They're known for removing excess oils, which is ideal for people with oily or acne-prone skin. Plus, who doesn't love playing with foam? The biggest downside to foam cleansers is that they often contain detergents, which is what makes them foam. Detergent tends to strip your skin of all oil (even the good kind), which you definitely don't want. Foam cleansers aren't my favorite, but to each their own I suppose. Just check the ingredients first to make sure it's free of sulfates.
- Using an *oil cleanser* may sound counterintuitive to the purpose of a cleanser (to *remove* oil), but it's simple science, really—oil

attracts oil. One of the main benefits of an oil cleanser is that it gently cleanses your skin without causing it to lose moisture. Some experts recommend "double cleansing," though, which involves using an oil cleanser first to dissolve stubborn makeup and then washing your face again with a regular cleanser.

Every skin type is different and what may work for your mom, sister, or friend might not work for you. If you're unsure of your skin type, consult with a dermatologist.

How often should I apply?: Twice a day

Toners

The next step in your skincare routine should be applying toner. People often choose to skip toners because there is a preconceived notion that they're too harsh and irritating. Luckily that's not the case anymore. Toners today are designed to be antiseptic and clarifying instead of drying. They're formulated to remove cleanser residue, salts, chlorines, and chemicals found in tap water that might pollute the skin (fun fact: chemicals that can be found in tap water essentially poison and age the skin), while also serving as a delivery system to receive the benefits of other products that will be layered on top. They often have moisturizing and antiaging benefits as well. Experts suggest wiping your toner in instead of just spraying it to completely remove any chemicals.

How often should I apply?: Once a day

Spot Treatments

If you're blessed with nearly flawless skin, then perhaps you can just skip this step, but if you're like me and use prescribed topicals, this is an important one. After your skin is prepped and clean, it's time to apply products that address specific concerns like acne, wrinkles, rosacea, and hyperpigmentation. These products tend to be more highly concentrated formulas that are designed to deliver benefits deep into the skin's layers—so it makes sense that they should be applied as closely to the skin as possible, right? Experts recommend allowing at least five minutes before layering your next product to ensure it doesn't inhibit the benefits of the medication.

How often should I apply?: Twice a day

Serums

Serums are often grouped together with spot treatments because they have a similar consistency and target specific concerns. Serums are highly concentrated, nutrient-dense treatments, so it's best to also keep these as close to the skin as possible—you take a daily vitamin everyday, so why shouldn't your skin? When it comes to selecting a serum, there is a wide variety to choose from based on ingredients and specific concerns. There are dozens of different serums that come from different vitamins, minerals, and oils, so I've chosen to elaborate on some of the most popular:

- *Vitamin C*: Vitamin C isn't just for your daily glass of orange juice. One of the most common ingredients in serums is vitamin C, because it performs a variety of functions including: stimulating new collagen, reducing fine lines and wrinkles, protecting the skin from pollutants, helping reduce discoloration, and protecting against UV exposure. Plus, since your skin doesn't produce vitamin C on its own, a topical serum is really the only way to reap those benefits. Your glowing skin will thank you later.

- *Peptides*: If you happen to remember anything from high school biology (first off, kudos), then maybe you would know that peptides are two amino acids linked together to form a bond. If you're looking to restore firmness, serums rich in peptides can boost collagen and elastin production—ideal for plumper-looking skin.

- *Omega-3*: You've heard of omega-3s before—they're in nutritious foods your doctor's always telling you to eat, like salmon and walnuts. Serums rich in essential oils and omega-3 fatty acids can help the skin to repair itself to ensure the barrier function is working at its best.

- *Hyaluronic Acid*: Hyaluronic acid isn't as scary as it sounds—it's likely in a variety of beauty products you already use because of its expert ability to retain moisture. You might be surprised to learn that it actually occurs naturally in connective tissue throughout the body and helps lubricate your joints. If it efficiently hydrates your insides, just imagine what wonders it will do for your skin.

- *Retinol*: As for the Holy Grail of serums, you've likely heard about the benefits of retinol (a derivative of vitamin A). Serums formulated with retinol can help regenerate cells and brighten your complexion to make it appear glowy and smooth—you know, that look you try to get with a pearlescent highlighter. Retinol was initially used to treat acne in the '60s, but doctors soon realized that it also helped with visible signs of aging. If used on a regular basis, it can improve skin texture, wrinkles, sun damage, enlarged pores, and acne—some studies have even shown that it can prevent skin cancer (yes, you still have to wear sunscreen). Retinol doesn't have many downsides, but, if it is used too frequently, your skin can start to become dry, red, and flaky. Over time, retinol can also thin the top layer of your skin, making it more susceptible to sun damage. Basically, with retinol more isn't more—a pea-sized drop goes a really long way. Nonetheless, retinols are widely accredited by dermatologists who insist that everyone should be using one and more importantly, you're never too young to start.

How often should I apply?: Twice a day

Moisturizers

When we're born, our skin automatically makes all the moisturizer it needs to be soft and healthy by creating sebum, a combination of oil and waxes. As we age, our skin's moisturizing abilities begin to slow, creating an imbalance (I guess it's true that youth is wasted on the young). When our skin doesn't have moisture, our complexion may appear dull, fine lines and wrinkles become more apparent, and the texture is downright flaky. Finding the right moisturizer is important but you need one that's going to fit your needs. Generally speaking, there are three different types of moisturizers:

- *Gels* disperse the ingredients via water, alcohol, or liquid fat base. They are typically the lightest and least greasy of moisturizers and often feel cool on the skin due to rapid evaporation. Gel moisturizers are ideal for people with oily skin because they contain the lowest level of emulsifiers, waxes, and oils. As a result, they replenish the skin without clogging your pores.
- *Lotions* are the product of dry powdered ingredients that have been dissolved in water. They're relatively light and absorb quickly into the skin to ensure you don't feel too greasy. Lotions are ideal for those with normal/combination skin because they have a high water content while providing some oil to help the skin retain hydration.
- *Creams* are the heaviest type of moisturizer because they consist of water and oil emulsion. Although they're the best at hydrating the skin, they often feel stickier and greasier than other lotions. Creams are ideal for those with dry skin because they create an occlusive layer around the skin that replaces the water and helps retain it. I wouldn't worry too much about it feeling greasy on your face, though—newer formulas are designed to absorb more quickly. Plus, if you've been dying for an excuse to splurge on Crème de la Mer (the 16.5-ounce jar is $2,160), here's me giving you permission.

If you know your skin type, I'm sure that sounds easy enough, but what if you want to use a face oil instead? Lately many women have been making the switch from moisturizer to face oil, but if you're not sure which is best for you, we have some tips:

- *Moisturizers*: Moisturizers are usually packed with a ton of ingredients that address multiple concerns, from acne to antiaging. A multitasking cream can help with brightening, firming, and plumping while the face oil's main function is to hydrate your skin. The waxes in moisturizers form an occlusive layer on the skin, which helps to hold in moisture, but they sometimes have a tendency to clog the pores and prevent the nutrients from penetrating the skin.
- *Oils*: Oils are ideal if your skin is dry but not sensitive. Since oils are rich in essential fatty acids, they moisturize your skin while repairing the outer barrier. But beware, not all oils are created equal: those containing saturated fats (like the beloved coconut oil) can clog your pores and cause acne. If you're going to choose an oil, you want one with a list of simple and natural ingredients. In fact, one of the reasons people are switching to face oils is because they create healthier skin without the exposure to chemicals, toxins, or harsh ingredients. Oils rich in fatty acids are required in our daily diet to stay healthy, so it only makes sense that they would have the same effect on our skin. Oils can also help with aging skin. As we get older, our skin produces less oil, which often results in wrinkles—a face oil adds it back through direct absorption and improves the lipid barrier function. Although typically recommended for dry skin, a face oil can work for a variety of skin types. If you're dry or blemished, the natural ingredients will help lock in moisture by creating a protective barrier while also cleansing pores. If you have oily skin, the natural ingredients in oils trick

your skin into thinking it already has enough, therefore shutting off sebum production and preventing shine. It's basically a win for everyone.

- *Tip*: no matter what the packaging says, it's best to apply oils after the shower while your skin is still damp. The moisture will help absorb the product better for all-day radiance.

How often should I apply?: Twice a day

Eye Cream

Eye cream used to be a distant worry—something you would see your mom or grandma applying to help eliminate wrinkles—but recently dermatologists have been recommending using it as a preventative measure starting as early as your twenties. But why can't I just use regular moisturizer? Eye creams are specifically formulated for the delicate skin around the eye, so they tend to be thicker. They also contain more oil than a regular moisturizer and have a lot of ingredients targeted to fix the eye's specific problems. Since the skin around the eye is more sensitive, it's more prone to a variety of issues like puffiness, dark circles, fine lines, and wrinkles. Plus, there are fewer oil glands around the eyes to help keep the skin naturally hydrated, so finding the right eye cream can help stave off a variety of concerns.

- *For puffiness*: Look for ingredients like caffeine or cucumber, which help reduce swelling. There's a reason why you always see cucumber eye treatments at spas and in classic movie scenes.
- *For dark circles*: Ingredients like vitamins C, vitamin K, and kojic acid can help with discoloration while peptides can help plump the skin. This means that even if you don't get a full night of sleep, there's still hope in the morning.
- *For wrinkles*: Any collagen-building ingredients like retinol should help smooth out fine lines. Buh-bye, crow's-feet.

Though you may not get the instant gratification like you would with a face mask or scrub, we can assure each application is making a difference that you'll be grateful for in the long run.

A tip: Experts suggest applying from the outside to the inside to counteract gravity's pull. Always apply eye cream with your ring finger using gentle dabbing instead of tugging. This will help prevent irritation, wrinkles, and sagging over time.

How often should I apply?: Twice a day

Sunscreen

It's a common myth that if it's winter, the sun has already set, or you're sitting inside all day, that there's no need for sunscreen—wrong! Just fifteen minutes outside each day is enough to cause damage. Sun exposure ages your skin and is really hard to reverse later in life. Experts recommend staying out of the sun as much as possible and applying an SPF 30 sunscreen daily. There are tons of oil-free sunscreens that provide protection without clogging your pores—mineral-based sunscreens are especially ideal for acne-prone skin. If you wear makeup on a regular basis, CC/BB creams and tinted moisturizers can also provide sun protection, but only if you put enough on. Whatever type of SPF you choose, make sure it's broad spectrum. You don't want those sun spots and wrinkles later in life.

How often should I apply?: Once every two to three hours (when in contact with the sun)

THE GOLDEN RULE A.K.A. HOW TO USE ALL OF THESE PRODUCTS AT THE SAME TIME

When you hear "The Golden Rule," you're likely to have flashbacks to your elementary school classroom, but the skincare world has a Golden Rule all its own: when layering products, always apply lightest to heaviest. Sure, "treating others the way you want to be treated" is important, but this one is essential if you want to get the most out of your skincare routine.

The reasoning is actually pretty simple—products that have low viscosity tend to have a smaller particle size, meaning they can more deeply penetrate your skin. Basically, products with a thinner consistency (toner, serum) will more effectively seep into your pores if they're applied first. After that, you work your way up to oils and creams—the thicker consistency products will help seal in the previous ones. Think of it like this: you wouldn't layer a thermal top over a chunky sweater, would you?

Another important tip is to let each product soak into the skin completely before adding another layer on top. This will ensure that you receive the maximum benefit from each product. After all, if you're going to spend over $70 on a serum, you want to get the most bang for your buck.

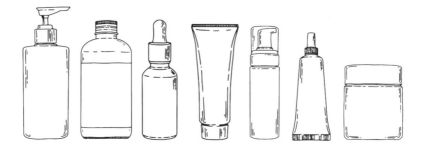

CHAPTER 2

Special Occasion

When it comes to the important events in our lives, I think it's safe to say we all want to look our best. For many people, a special occasion may be a prom, wedding, or important job interview, while for others, "it's a Tuesday" is a good enough excuse. Of course, when we know that photos will be taken, it heightens the stakes a bit. We idealize what the day will be like—and glowing skin is often a part of it. After all, we all want something brag-worthy to show our grandchildren; I want mine to ask, "Was Grandma a literal angel, mom?" "Nope, that's just microdermabrasion and a killer highlight, son."

Facials, laser treatments, and sweat protection are all a part of your big day, too. What masks should I be using? What's Fraxel? How far in advance should I be starting these procedures? Will my skin ever glow like Halle Berry's circa *ever* (there's no way she's fifty-two)? I've included both the normal and crazy options—I'm pretty sure the only one I omitted was Gwyneth's "bee sting" facial and that's only because I don't want to be liable for someone else's hospital bill.

When to Get A Facial

Congrats! Your big day is coming up. You might be thinking to yourself, *I have plenty of time!,* but in the skincare world, it's better to get an early start. Ask any qualified aesthetician and she'll likely tell you that regular facials should be started at least six months prior to your event—combined with a consistent and quality skincare routine, of course. There are a few reasons for this. First of all, you don't want to try a new treatment right before your big day, only to find out that your skin didn't react so well—some facials can be abrasive and leave temporary redness. Secondly, the effects of facials will often magnify the more frequently you do them—most experts would suggest a facial once a month. Before you know it, your skin will look flawless just in time for those angelic wedding photos.

If you're considering photofacials, microdermabrasion, acid peels, or laser hair removal, you'll also want at least a six-month start in order to see positive results. Lastly, if you're considering self-tanners or spray tans, I would suggest experimenting at least three months prior. Let's just say I had a former coworker who made that mistake a week before her wedding.

Types of Facials

Now you're probably wondering, *but what type of facial is right for me?* Perhaps you have acne or sun-damaged skin. Maybe you're looking to contour your face. If you're preparing for a wedding, I can assume you like diamonds and may therefore want to consider a facial with some crushed up bling.

You'll need to find a trusted spa as well since most facials are nearly impossible to do at home (correctly, at least). How much will it cost? Well, it varies depending on the length and quality of the treatment. Thirty-minute classic facials can sometimes be as little as $50 while ninety-minute niche ones can be as much as $700 (or more). Generally speaking, the average facial costs about $80 to $90, or as I'd like to say *almost one monthly MetroCard in New York*—you'll want the walk anyways to show off your new radiant skin.

If this feels overwhelming, don't worry. It's about to feel simple. Here's an extensive list that includes everything from standard options to snail slime.

Let's start with the microcurrent facial since that seems to be a very popular choice these days for brides-to-be.

During a **Microcurrent Facial**, a set of skinny metal wands is used to emit a mild electrical current that stimulates the skin and facial muscles to create a facelift effect. This technology has been used for over a century to heal tissue damage and other injuries because it speeds up cell production and repair. The reason it's so popular is because the results are noticeable (and impressive) after just one treatment. After a single session, it will contour the face, improve skin tone, reduce wrinkles and dark circles, and promote blood circulation and collagen production. Oh, and it's completely painless. With modern technology and short attention spans, we've become a society that wants things immediately—and this procedure does just that. Plus, since there's no extraction involved, your skin won't have any of the redness and irritation that can come from traditional facials. Some experts even say it's safe to get the day before a wedding. Plus, one treatment is said to take up to seven years off your face. Talk about a glow-up!

Classic Facial: consists of steaming, deep cleansing, exfoliation, extractions, a lymph massage, toner, and moisturizer. It's the standard go-to facial that tends to be suited for just about everyone. I'm sure you've seen videos of it before. Your friends have probably gotten them, too. You can't really go wrong with this one.

Oxygen Facial: a machine sprays atomized moisturizers onto the skin using a stream of pressurized oxygen that's infused with vitamins, minerals, essential nutrients, and botanical extracts. It hydrates skin instantly, making the face appear smoother and fuller. Celebrities like Madonna swear by it because it temporarily diminishes the tiny imperfections that would be visible on HD TV. It has many benefits, some of which include: boosting collagen production, speeding up cell turnover, and healing acne. Brides love it because it allows your foundation to go on smoothly.

Hydrating Facial: *hydrates* your skin with moisture to diminish fine lines and create a dewy complexion. The process is similar to that of a classic facial but usually includes humectant-rich products and masks.

Brightening Facial: involves a combination of masks, enzyme peels, and acid treatments to remove dead skin and buildup. It'll not only improve your skin tone, but also help reduce the appearance of sun damage and age spots. As the name implies, you'll be left with dewy, glowing clear skin.

HydraFacial: the only hydradermabrasion procedure that combines cleansing, exfoliation, extraction, hydration, and antioxidant protection simultaneously. Okay, let's break that down. Basically, instead of using harsh exfoliants like traditional dermabrasion, it vacuums out pores while simultaneously infusing them with potent actives. The result is clear and moisturized skin with absolutely no irritation. It also helps improve the appearance of wrinkles, enlarged pores, acne, and hyperpigmentation.

Microdermabrasion Facial: now that "hydradermabrasion" has been thrown into the mix, I may as well address microdermabrasion, the noninvasive form of "dermabrasion." This type of facial buffs away the layers of dead skin by using a pressurized jet with micronized crystals and then vacuuming away the dead skin cells. Like most facials, it can help with pigmentation, fine lines, and acne scars.

Decongesting Facial: is designed to clear out clogged pores and eliminate blackheads. Although gentle acid peels are sometimes used, the facial almost exclusively focuses on extractions—so if you're like me and struggle with acne (or find intense satisfaction from watching Dr. Pimple Popper videos), this one might be for you. Your skin might be slightly irritated right after the treatment but they should never hurt or cause scarring when performed correctly.

LED Facial (Color Light Therapy): uses wavelengths of UV-free LED light that claim to treat a variety of issues. Each color serves a different purpose. For example, blue light destroys acne-causing bacteria while red light stimulates collagen production and promotes circulation. The good news is it's painless and noninvasive. Bad news is that it often takes several and consistent sessions to start noticing dramatic results.

Lymphatic Massage Facial: a soothing massage that uses gentle brushing motions to move fluid out of tissues and into your lymph nodes where bacteria, viruses, and other harmful organisms are destroyed. In addition to protecting against pathogens, it reduces swelling in the face—perfect for those looking for a more contoured jawline or reduced eye puffiness.

Firming and Contouring Facial: incorporates massaging techniques to firm and sculpt your face. The effects are similar to that of a microcurrent facial, only it doesn't use any devices. Not everyone finds this intense treatment to be super relaxing, though, so I probably wouldn't recommend it to unwind right before your big day.

Acupuncture Facial: dermal needles are inserted approximately one millimeter into the frown lines, forehead, and crow's-feet to improve circulation and increase natural collagen production. I probably don't need to tell you this, but acupuncture needles don't hurt.

Aromatherapy Facial: solely uses aromatherapy oil (and sometimes steam and a facial peel) to help create healthy, glowing, and moisturized skin. The essential oils have soothing properties that can also help eliminate acne. Plus, it'll also help you relax your mind for your big day.

Paraffin Facial: involves covering your face with a protective gauze mask and warm paraffin wax. The paraffin's warmth opens your pores and allows moisturizers to penetrate more easily. When removed, it takes old skin cells with it, leaving the skin silky smooth. This holistic approach has been around since the Roman empire and is still loved today for its ability to reduce wrinkles, moisturize your face, and relax you. I'm sure you've seen this facial in TV shows and movies.

Fruit Facial: use acids derived from fruit to deeply scrub the skin and remove blackheads. It's also believed to stimulate collagen, improve skin texture, and reduce wrinkles. Plus, the vitamin C found in fruits can help lighten scarring and blemishes. Although it might smell good, don't eat the product after using it.

Diamond File Facial: involves a stainless-steel tool that has actual crushed diamonds on one side that polish the skin without damaging it. Sounds gimmicky, I know. But if Marilyn Monroe taught us anything, it's that "diamonds are a girl's best friend"—and as gemstone treatments go, we promise this one is more effective than jade eggs. That's because diamonds contain trace elements and when applied topically, stimulate cell turnover and fight free radicals. Your skin will feel brand new and have fewer dark spots.

Gold Facial: while we're on the topic of diamonds, we may as well delve into gold. A gold facial involves all of the steps in a classic one, but ends with a gold face mask—usually either 24-karat gold leaf or colloidal gold. It's known to improve circulation, remove toxins, and lighten pigmentation, making it ideal for those with dull skin. They can be pricey but it's your day so you may as well indulge.

Fire & Ice Facial: using elements of heat and cold, this facial brightens, smooths, and tightens skin. The protocol varies from spa to spa but all of them incorporate heat to increase blood flow and then a cold treatment to reduce inflammation. Many Hollywood stars use it to get a glowing complexion for a red-carpet appearance.

Vampire Facial: is a combination of microdermabrasion followed by a mask of platelet-rich plasma (PRP), which helps boost your skin's cell turnover. The PRP contains platelets which have a higher concentration of growth factors. In layman's terms, tiny holes are poked into your skin and injected with your own blood to stimulate cell turnover. It can help increase collagen, reduce scars, and minimize wrinkles. My guess is you've already seen this trendy treatment on one of the Kardashians' Instagram accounts. It can be very painful if they don't numb you beforehand, though. Fun fact: it doubles as a gory Halloween costume.

Snail Facial: is exactly what it sounds like. Live snails are applied to the face to work their magic. This technique actually dates back to ancient Greece where Hippocrates used it to heal burns and wounds. The snail's mucus contains proteins, antioxidants, and—everyone's favorite—hyaluronic acid, which help rejuvenate the skin. It's a bit pricey and probably not for everyone.

Masks

Okay so maybe you're a low-maintenance bride and prefer to stick to inexpensive and easy solutions. Perhaps you're simply looking to supplement your facials and skin care routine. Might I suggest the wonderful world of face masks? I'm sure you've seen them in your local drugstore, Sephora, or perhaps even made them as a teenager with your friends at sleepovers—bananas, honey, and baking soda, anyone? It may be hard to believe that a simple ten-minute treatment can make all that much of a difference, but it can. Here's why: face masks contain a higher concentration of the active ingredients found in your favorite lotions and cleansers, which is why your complexion looks instantly better after taking one off. Basically, they deliver dramatic results in a short period of time, making them an important part of preparing for your special occasion.

Now I know what you're thinking: there are tons of different types of face masks. Which ones should I use and when should I use them?

Six to nine months before (an important time frame for preparation) is a good time to experiment with peel-off masks. If you need a visual, just imagine the opening scene in the 2000 film *American Psycho*, or that black charcoal mask challenge that vent viral on YouTube a couple of years ago. You simply apply the product on your face, wait for it

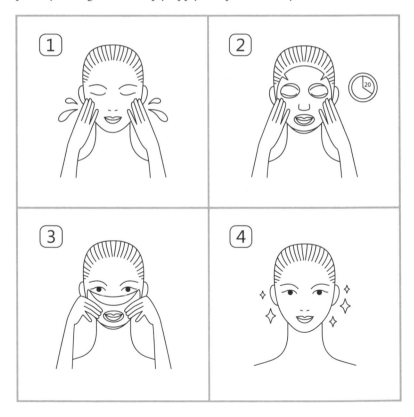

to dry, and then gently peel it off. This will help rid your skin of any sebum or debris from your pores. After you remove it and rinse your face, you'll notice brighter and tighter skin.

Three to five months before is ideal for using exfoliating masks. Exfoliating masks are great for all skin types because they help remove dead skin cells, leaving your face feeling fresh and smooth. Since it gets deep into your pores, it allows better absorption for moisturizers and other treatments. Once you apply the mask onto your face, gently massage it in a circular motion, let it sit for a few minutes, and then rinse with warm water. Be sure not to use them too frequently, though—I wouldn't recommend more than once a week.

One to three months before is a great time for gel masks. That's because the gel soothes and cools the skin to help repair and replenish, making it ideal for those with dry or sensitive skin. It will definitely help with any dryness, redness, or irritation so that you're camera-ready for your big day. Simply apply the gel to your face, let it sit for a few minutes, and rinse with warm water. Pretty easy, no?

The **last month** before is perfect for clay masks. Clay masks have tons of benefits such as clearer pores and brighter skin. Although they're ideal for normal to oily skin, they're great for all skin types. As the clay tightens, it soaks up all the skin's natural oils and anything clogging the pores will be brought to the surface like a magnet to steel. Not only is it an all-natural approach that's been around for centuries, but it's gentle and won't have any negative side effects. If you're looking for other benefits, it's antimicrobial and can therefore help heal skin issues like psoriasis and eczema. It also oxygenates the cells, shrinks pores, reduces inflammation, and regulates sebum production. After you apply the mask, let it sit until completely dry (your skin will feel super tight and might even tingle), and then remove it with warm water.

As you probably noticed, most of those masks decreased in intensity and risk—you don't want to experiment with a new exfoliating mask the day before a wedding or graduation, I promise. In fact, if your skin is dry or you're craving an extra boost, I would recommend using a sheet mask on your big day. A sheet mask is concentrated with a serum and will help replenish your skin for a last-minute surge of hydration.

Lasers and Dermatologic Procedures

Okay, I know we took it down a notch with masks, but now we're actually going to take it up again with lasers and dermatologic procedures. There are *so* many different options out there. I'm pretty sure there are more dermatologic procedures out there than there are waterproof mascaras . . . and that's saying a lot. There are different options for different needs, and of course, time frames.

TO REDUCE WRINKLES:

Let's dive into the most popular procedure: **Botox**. I'm pretty sure we're all familiar with the treatment, but more and more people are using it for preventative measures. It's not uncommon for a bride in her twenties to receive her first Botox treatment right before her big day. I've said it once, I'll say it 500 more times: who doesn't want porcelain-smooth skin for their photos? Nothing is better than Botox to ease lines around the eyes, forehead, and eyebrows. How does it work? Botox (a purified protein) paralyzes the muscles in the desired areas. It takes a few days to kick in but usually lasts a few months.

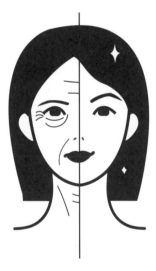

Bonus points: it can even be used for overly active sweat glands to reduce severe underarm perspiration so you don't have to worry about pit stains on your expensive gown.

Time Frame: One to two months before.

If Botox isn't your thing, there are tons of alternatives on the market right now:

Juvéderm: a gel made from hyaluronic acid (a natural complex sugar found in the body) that temporarily reduces wrinkles from the nose to the corners of the mouth, a.k.a. nasolabial folds.
Lasts: Six months.

Voluma (also a part of the Juvéderm line): is designed to add volume under the skin's surface to lift and contour the cheeks. Voluma also contains hyaluronic acid.
Lasts: up to two years.

Restylane: composed of hyaluronic acid and is used for fine lines and moderate wrinkles. It's also one of the first widely used fillers.
Lasts: Four to six months.

Sculptra: a filler composed of synthetic poly-L-lactic acid that's injected under the skin and into the fatty layers to replace lost volume, sculpt, and reduce sagging.
Lasts: Two years.

Radiesse: calcium-based synthetic filler that's used for deep skin folds and wrinkles to help plump the skin. The benefits continue by stimulating your body's own natural collagen—pretty cool, huh? It can also be used for scars and to fill out depressions and angles in the nose.
Lasts: Two years.

Perlane: composed of hyaluronic acid that has a larger particle size than other fillers, which allows for a deeper injection into the skin. It's used for softening wrinkles, acne scars, facial folds, and even lip injections.
Lasts: Three to nine months.

Evolence: derived from pig collagen and is one of the newest fillers on the market. It works best for softening medium-depth skin folds and wrinkles such as those from the nose to corner of the mouth. It can also be used on other areas, though, such as the lips, nose, and cheeks.

Lasts: One to two years.

SilkPeel®: is designed to improve the appearance of skin. Similar to microdermabrasion, it removes the outer layers of skin with exfoliation, however it also uses various serums that are designed to target specific problems. It can be used on virtually any part of the body to treat acne, minimize wrinkles, reduce sun spots, and hydrate skin. It's not as intense as chemical peels, laser skin resurfacing, or photofacials—plus, it's more affordable. Results are immediately visible.

Lasts: Up to six weeks.

Ultherapy: uses ultrasound energy to lift and tighten the skin naturally, specifically improving the appearance of lines and wrinkles on the décolletage—if you're wearing a low neckline, you know how important this is! Plus, it's the only noninvasive procedure that's FDA-cleared, if that sort of thing is important to you.

Lasts: Anywhere from one to five years but it really depends on each individual's own natural collagen production. You'll notice results after three to twelve months.

TO REDUCE SUN SPOTS AND DISCOLORATION:

Fraxel: microscopic laser beams penetrate deep into the skin to create tiny wounds, which trigger the body's natural response to create collagen and elastin. It's best for sun spots, fine lines, and sagging, but regardless, you'll end up with tighter, fresher, and younger-looking skin, making it especially popular for brides over thirty. It can be somewhat painful, though, so dermatologists often use a topical anesthesia before the treatment. Results aren't usually visible until two or three months after the treatment.

Time Frame: Four months before.

Clear & Brilliant: uses the same type of laser as Fraxel, but at a lower intensity, which means it's virtually pain-free. One session removes superficial sun damage but multiple treatments can fight deeper damage. Either way, your skin will look more radiant and well-rested. You'll see results immediately, but it's still recommended that you book an appointment at least three to six weeks before your special occasion. You'll likely have at least twelve to twenty-four hours of redness and swelling.

Time Frame: One month before.

Q-Switched: unlike Fraxel and Clear & Brilliant, it uses a YAG laser which targets melanin (dark spots) on the surface of the skin to eliminate pigment discoloration: sun spots, age spots, freckles. After the treatment, each spot will turn into a scab and then heal after five to seven days. The same technology is also used to get rid of tattoos, so if you're looking to do that before your big day, it's a one-stop shop.

Time Frame: Three months out.

V-Beam: is a type of pulse dye laser that's designed to eliminate redness (whether it's just a bit of irritation or all-over rosacea). It's ideal for those with fairer skin. The more severe the redness, the more treatments you'll need. You'll be even redder than usual after the treatment (oh, the irony) but it will go down after a week.

Time Frame: At least two weeks before.

Intense Pulsed Light: a concentrated flash of light passes through the top skin layer and into the deeper layer to help improve redness from rosacea and broken capillaries. Not only will you have an even complexion, but you'll also notice that your makeup goes on a lot smoother.

Time Frame: Five months out.

TO REDUCE ACNE:

I think most of us would agree that one of the most frustrating things to happen to your skin before a big day is acne. For some, that might be the occasional pimple but for others, acne can mean several breakouts, of several types of blemishes, in several places. If you eat healthy, exercise on a regular basis, and have tried every topical cleanser and cream imaginable, it might be time to resort to dermatologic treatments.

Isolaz: is a procedure that uses a new technology called Photopneumatics, which blends a vacuum with a painless laser. The vacuum extracts oil from the pores while the laser eliminates the skin's bacterial content. Eighty-five percent of patients report improvement in their acne, but it can also be used to remove unwanted hair and sun damage. Plus, it's painless and has very few side effects.

Time Frame: One month out.

Cortisone Shot: is a quick injection of steroid that will fight both inflammation and acne instantly. Since it'll eliminate a pimple in twenty-four to forty-eight hours, it's perfect for any last-minute blemishes that may arise before your big day.

Time Frame: One to two days before.

CHEMICAL PEELS:

Whenever I think of a chemical peel, I can't help but recall Samantha's unfortunate treatment the day of Carrie's book launch party. The large black hat with the veil looked great of course, but the comparison to "beef carpaccio" still haunts me to this day. All of this is a long-winded way of saying I've never tried a chemical peel, but I've heard good things post-*Sex and the City*.

Chemical peels have ingredients like AHAs and BHAs and are a bit harsher than enzyme peels, which have ingredients like pumpkin, pineapple, and papaya. Both will remove dead skin cells and result in a healthy glow, but the former will cost you some temporary discomfort. You'll need at *least* six weeks between your appointment and your big day because you don't want to risk any redness. The process works for most skin types, but seems to work best on those with fair skin and light hair.

Time Frame: Three months out.

LASER HAIR REMOVAL—BODY & FACE:

I truly can't think of a more useful cosmetic treatment than laser hair removal. After five to six sessions, the hair is gone—well, usually. Sometimes you need touchups after a few years, but it's mostly permanent. That means the effects will last long after your big day. The number one laser request from brides is armpit hair removal, but I say, "Why stop there?" Laser your legs, bikini line, sideburns, lower back, etc. Of course, I embrace a woman's choice to keep her hair (a choice I often select myself), but the convenience of not having to shave is liberating.

A laser works by selective photothermolysis—a.k.a. a light targets a specific color in your follicles, which results in hair removal. Since you need at least four to six weeks between each session because of hair growth cycles, most experts recommend starting six to twelve months before your big day. When I did laser hair removal on my upper legs, I deliberately started treatments in the winter. First off, your skin is highly sensitive in between treatments and can easily burn or scar when exposed to UV rays. Secondly, I wanted to be smooth just in time for swimwear season. Granted, I wasn't preparing for a special occasion, but planning is key!

It's also important to know that you can't wax or thread in between treatments. Shaving only. Oh yeah, and another problem with lasers: unfortunately, most lasers don't work well on blonde or red hair, or people with darker skin. The laser literally has trouble differentiating color and therefore does not always do its job correctly. Fortunately for me, I'm very pale and have thick, dark brown leg hair, making me an ideal candidate. But, it is incredibly frustrating that laser technology hasn't evolved enough to be more advanced and inclusive. If laser hair removal isn't your thing, there are some other alternatives.

Time Frame: Six months out.

ELECTROLYSIS:

The first major difference between laser hair removal and electrolysis is that electrolysis can be used on anyone, regardless of their skin or hair color. Woohoo! That's because it attacks the follicle itself and not the pigment in the hair. Generally speaking, electrolysis is also better at *permanently* removing hair. Unlike laser hair removal, electrolysis is also backed by the FDA.

One major downfall of electrolysis is that it's usually best for smaller areas on the body, like toes and upper lips. That's because the electronic needle used is inserted into each individual hair root, making it much more time consuming. It usually also requires more treatments than laser hair removal. Therefore, even though each electrolysis treatment is cheaper, it'll eventually add up to possibly being more expensive than five or six pricey laser treatments. Oh yeah, and electrolysis tends to also be more painful. I personally found laser hair removal to be relatively painful (even with the numbing cream they gave me) so if they say electrolysis is more painful, I don't want to know what it's like . . . especially since every follicle has to experience the wrath. Ouch. Oh yeah, and scarring is more likely with it, too.

DERMAPLANING:

In case you've never heard of it, dermaplaning is a method of exfoliation that involves using a surgical #10 blade (yes, the same ones used by surgeons) to gently scrape off the top layer of dead skin cells and facial hair in order to reveal a smoother, brighter complexion. Though a #10 scalpel may seem intimidating, it's completely painless.

Dermaplaning is great for all skin types, except for those with cystic acne. And contrary to popular belief, your hair won't grow back thicker or darker. It usually only takes about thirty minutes per procedure and costs anywhere from $100 to $300. There are also no side effects or downtime. Unfortunately, I think this is one of those treatments that becomes addictive so I suppose the cost could add up. But if you're just looking for smooth skin before your big day, this could be a great option.

You've probably seen your friends and favorite bloggers start using it recently, but it's been a favorite in the entertainment industry for a while because it eliminates the peach fuzz that can now be seen with harsh camera lighting and HD televisions. It also allows for greater penetration of skincare products and a smoother canvas for makeup—perfect for photos on your big day. I personally have always considered not shaving your face to be one of the *perks* of being a woman, but to each their own. I've actually heard really great things about it.

I've also seen videos lately of a lot of women doing it themselves at home, but I would recommend a specialist. A face scar before your big day usually isn't a great look.

Miscellaneous

Body Wrap: is all about relaxation so if you're super stressed in the days leading up to a big event, indulge. Select a full-body exfoliation before the body wrap so that your skin absorbs the ingredients. Plus, there are different kinds on the market including ones for slimming, detoxifying, and calming.

Time Frame: A few days before.

Products to Use for Flawless Skin and Sweat Protection

Okay so you've been preparing for the last six months with facials, lasers, and masks. You have the perfect outfit picked out. You know how you want to wear your hair. But wait, what about makeup? I'm sure if you're reading this, you're already relatively knowledgeable about makeup. But you want to make sure your makeup stays intact on such an important day—through all the sweat, tears, environmental changes, laughter . . . I don't know what's happening on your big day, but you want to look flawless.

We already touched on armpit Botox and spray tans, but I feel the need to reiterate because they will both really help with sweat protection and glowing skin respectively. I by no means think you need either. In fact, I've never gotten either in my life. But they are really popular among brides, so perhaps it's something to consider. Botox minimizes and blocks out the body's sweat glands, for anywhere from six months to a year. Essentially, it blocks the nerves from reaching the sweat glands and decreases the chemical reaction.

Now for the fun stuff: makeup! Everyone wants to glow these days without being (or looking) sweaty . . . such a fine line, no? Let's start with the "glow" part. Before putting on their makeup, most women opt for a moisturizer. The easiest way to radiate is to choose a moisturizer that has an illuminating effect. It will help your face catch the light from every angle. Luckily, they're pretty popular right now so you can find them at pretty much every drug and makeup store. Over that, I would suggest a satin-finish foundation. Foundation tends to cake sometimes—even makeup Kween Kylie Jenner admitted that in one of her interviews recently. Satin has luminosity, though, and makes the skin look pretty without looking glittery. It's essentially designed to evoke the dewiness of natural skin, unlike matte formulas.

Okay, now let's address the "sweaty" part. Before you put on your foundation, I would apply an oil-free sunscreen and matte primer. The oil-free part will prevent breakouts and shiny skin while still protecting you from harmful rays. The matte primer will prevent foundation from sliding off your face, which I know sounds like hyperbole but if you've ever seen it, you know. It's not a pretty sight or comfortable experience. Once you're all done applying your makeup (foundations, concealers, powders, shadows, etc.), finish off the whole look with a matte setting spray. Most feature temperature-control technology that actually lowers the temperature of your makeup in the heat to keep it from getting shiny. Pretty advanced if you ask me. Oh, and don't worry. You won't ruin your makeup by setting it with spray.

If you're really that worried about sweat, put on some waterproof mascara and sweep your hair up so that it's up off your neck. Oh yeah, and deodorant. But I felt I shouldn't even need to mention that . . . right? Try a clinical strength if you're worried about pit stains but don't feel the need to get armpit Botox.

CHAPTER 3
Nightly Rituals

What is it about having a nightly routine that's so satisfying and calming? After a long day of work, running off to yoga, picking up the kids from soccer, cooking dinner, etc., it's nice having a moment to take care of yourself. It's therapeutic, in a way. You're in control for once and giving your skin some much-needed TLC. I think of my evening routine as being a bit pared down, but if I'm being honest with myself, it's probably not. I've gotten better, though! I now only use four skincare products after my evening shower—two for my face, one for my upper body, and one for my legs to minimize redness after shaving. Plus, eye cream and hand lotion and, okay, I'm not low-maintenance.

If you've ever been sucked into the YouTube beauty world, you would also know that nighttime routines are a big thing. I've watched hundreds of them . . . hundreds. I wish I could say, "It was for my job! I had to!" But the reality is, I find them super intriguing and addicting. I love learning about other people's rituals and what products they're using. "Maybe if I copy her, I can have glowing skin like she does," I say to myself. "Maybe I'll also have her cool job, killer wardrobe, and beautiful apartment." That's how it works, right? I know I'm not alone because each video can rack up millions of views. Accounts like *Into the Gloss* might showcase a new It-Girl for every video, but YouTubers like Olivia Jade have done several nighttime routine videos (eight, to be exact) with each racking up views in the hundreds of thousands (sometimes millions). And if it also happens to incorporate ASMR . . . don't get me started. I could watch those for days at a time.

You would think that since the YouTube and beauty world is filled with videos, articles, and products for nightly rituals that it would be comprehensive, right? But for some reason there are still so many unanswered questions. Is beauty sleep a real thing? Are night creams a scam? But what if I actually *am* low-maintenance? A lot of confusion and conflicting evidence can leave us feeling a bit uneasy. Let's explore the elusive world of nightly rituals.

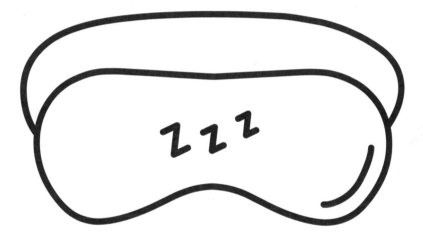

Beauty Sleep

I should probably preface this by saying that there is a lot of contradicting opinions on many of these topics. Some dermatologists might say yes, others might say no. Research might show one thing while testimonials say otherwise. I've tried to incorporate both sides of the argument while hopefully giving you the most accurate consensus. If you don't like my opinion, then hopefully you have enough information to form your own.

"Beauty sleep." Is it just me or do you automatically think of Sleeping Beauty: her flushed skin, bright eyes, that off-the-shoulder gown . . .

Anyway, I'm sure you've heard the term many times in your life. Perhaps your grandmother said it because she truly believes it works, or maybe your mom said it to trick you into going to bed early as a kid.

According to a study conducted last year by Royal Society Open Science, "beauty sleep" is very much a real thing. In fact, the study shows that people who get less sleep appear less attractive to others—ouch. While a couple of sleepless nights aren't enough to make someone look "ugly," consistently lacking sleep can result in dark eye circles, puffy eyelids, sallow skin, and tired faces—which can apparently make you less approachable, too. Researchers asked a group of students to get two consecutive nights of good sleep and then two consecutive nights of only four hours of sleep. Strangers were asked to rank the tiredness, attractiveness, and approachability of these students in photos after both the good and bad sleep sessions. Not surprisingly, the "lack of sleep" photos suffered. It makes sense from an evolutionary standpoint. An "unhealthy-looking" face could potentially signal to another person that you have a disease. And we all want our partners to be attractive and energetic, right? We should be more evolved than this by now, but whatever. I guess the silver lining is that if you want to make more friends, just get more sleep? Or be nice and give people free compliments. "You look well-rested and eye bag–free today." Let me know how that goes.

Generally speaking, a good night's sleep is always a good idea for your skin, but some experts disagree on the long-term impacts. Lack of sleep *can* increase dark circles, wrinkles, etc., but it's usually only temporary. That's because lack of sleep doesn't impact actual cell turnover. When the body is tired, it increases the production of cortisol to give you an extra boost of energy to stay awake. Unfortunately, cortisol also increases the volume of blood vessels—the cause of dark circles. I'm sure you've noticed it happen to you. You stay up late a few nights in a row and you're bound to see dark, puffy eyes. Then the weekend comes and you finally get to catch up on your sleep deficit—you wake up with skin that looks healthy and radiates brighter than a Rembrandt painting. "I'm never going to let myself miss out on sleep again," you tell yourself.

While your skin can survive on little sleep before eventually bouncing back, I still stress the importance of sleep for every bodily function. Because it's a chain reaction, isn't it? If your body feels run down, your skin will, too. And then it becomes a vicious cycle. And before you know it you have blemishes, puffy eyes, and dull skin—or what some people would call a regular Monday morning.

Night Creams

I believe it was the great Socrates who posed the age-old question: "Do night creams really work?" Just kidding. He was too busy creating eponymous methods and metaphysical hypotheses. But the beauty industry has been asking it for what feels like decades. In case you don't know, a night cream is a moisturizer that's marketed for evening. It's often thicker and more expensive . . . but we'll get to the differences shortly.

Considering there is so much skepticism around night creams, there sure are a lot on the market. I went on both Sephora's and Ulta's websites to try to figure out what kind of words beauty brands are using

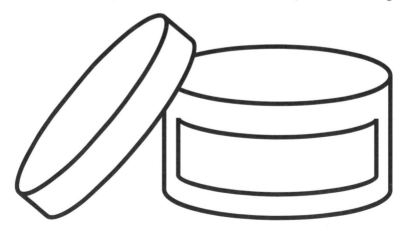

to target consumers. I found it interesting that the adjectives, verbs, and nouns they use are incredibly descriptive and strongly associated with medicinal qualities. Another thing I noticed (which I doubt means anything but is interesting nonetheless) is that they use *a lot* of *r* words: restorative, renewal, regenerating, resurgence, repairing, reform, recovery, radiance, replenisher, resurfacing, revitalizing, recharging. You feel rejuvenated—got another—just *looking* at them.

DAY CREAMS VS. NIGHT CREAMS

The main difference when it comes to daytime versus nighttime products is this: daytime is about protection from the environment, nighttime is about repairing. Daytime moisturizers have a lighter consistency and often contain SPF as well as free-radical-fighting antioxidants (like vitamin C). The lighter formula also makes them ideal for layering under makeup. Nighttime moisturizers are formulated to make skin soft and supple. Your skin loses a lot of water while you sleep, so nighttime products are specifically formulated to combat that. They have a much thicker consistency than day creams, which can help the absorption of the other vitamins and ingredients found in your serums and oils. Night creams are so thick that they actually aren't aesthetically pleasing enough to wear during the day and are nearly impossible to wear under makeup.

DO I NEED THEM?

But that probably still doesn't answer your question: Do I *need* them or are they just a marketing ploy? Once again, contradictions galore.

Some experts say that you don't need them or that they're just a gimmick. Here's what skeptics have argued: As long as you're using a moisturizer, that's all that matters. A moisturizer for night is one that simply doesn't have sunscreen. They're just expensive moisturizers that don't provide any added benefit. Moisturizers don't have to be greasy or heavy to get the job done because it's a myth that heavier formulations work better on wrinkles. There's no magic in the night that warrants using a special moisturizer because the skin doesn't have any special processes that it doesn't do during the day. Although there are physiological differences in the skin while lying down, there are no studies that correlate stages of sleep with skin activity. Be critical when it comes to marketing tactics because brands use special terms to sell their products. Although they are a bit thicker, found in smaller jars, and at a higher price point, there are no specific ingredients in night creams that function differently depending on the time of day, because . . . ingredients don't know what time of day it is.

Okay. Phew. That was a long explanation. Now on to the believers: Some ingredients do their job more effectively when used at certain times. Skin uses the night to repair itself from damages of the day (sun exposure, stress, pollution) and night creams are designed to enhance that natural process with products that accelerate regrowth (stem cell simulators, retinol, and DNA-repairing enzymes).

Okay, so the positives list was kind of short. While I agree that night creams aren't specifically formulated to have magical powers at night, I do think that they are formulated with some benefits that you would only want at night (i.e., thick consistency, no sunscreen, restorative qualities). I think that as long as you're informed about what you're buying, there's no harm in indulging. If a night cream makes you feel extra hydrated and refreshed—my last *r* word, I promise—then go for it. But if you're spending upward of a hundred dollars for a magical potion, you're likely out of luck.

IS SKIN DIFFERENT AT NIGHT?

Okay so now we know the differences between day and night cream but is my skin actually different at night? And the experts say . . . more discrepancies. Oy.

We already touched upon it in the previous section, but the skeptics that argue against night cream are the same ones who believe the skin doesn't function any differently at night. They believe that our skin functions the same at night as it does during the day so there's no magical product that could work specifically for night.

On the contrary, though, there's overwhelming evidence that proves otherwise. According to many studies, skin function *does* change at night. Skin's detox enzymes are released, cell division increases, mitochondrial energy is renewed, and DNA repair is active. Not to mention the fact that water content in the cells is at its lowest (meaning you lose moisture) and the skin's protective barrier function is decreased for better permeability of products. It's also been proven that new skin cells *do* grow faster while you sleep. Basically, our cells go into overdrive to repair damage from the day. Our blood vessels dilate, which allows an increased flow of nutrients and oxygen to the skin, which helps stimulate the removal of toxins. In the process, collagen also regenerates thanks to increased melatonin and lower cortisol levels. If you're the type of person that needs scientific backing: cell regeneration allegedly peaks between 11:00 p.m. and 4:00 a.m.—sounds legit, no?

If you're looking for a middle-ground answer, the process of cell turnover isn't much different depending on the time of day, but it does happen at a higher rate at night. Our body has a twenty-four-hour circadian rhythm, meaning that these processes are happening all the time but occur maximally at different times of the day—so no worries, skin doesn't stop repairing itself when your alarm clock goes off at 6:00 a.m.

WHAT NIGHT PRODUCTS ARE RIGHT FOR ME?

Okay, now that you know all the pros and cons of night products and you've decided to buy one, here's how to know which ones are right for you:

- **If you're acne-prone**: opt for a purifying cream.

- **If your skin is dry**: rich, creamy textures . . . I'm giving you another reason to indulge on Crème de La Mer (or as I call it, *two months of rent*).
- **If you're in your twenties**: choose a night cream that allows the skin to repair damage from sun exposure and stress. Now's the time to find one of those *r*-word products. Look for ones with stellar reviews.
- **If you're in your thirties or older**: choose an anti-wrinkle cream to slow aging and brighten your complexion.

We already went over these in chapter one, but here are some ingredients to look for:

- **Retinols**: reduce the appearance of wrinkles and dark spots. They're also best for night because they can deactivate and irritate with sun exposure.
- **Peptides**: stimulate the growth of new cells and shedding of dead cells.
- **Vitamin C**: helps fight free radical damage and stimulate new cell growth. It's great at night because it can be broken down by sun exposure.
- **AHA, BHA**: exfoliate the skin to get rid of dead skin cells. It's also best at night because they increase sensitivity to the sun.

Low-Maintenance(ish) Night Routine

Okay, so maybe you really are low-maintenance. Maybe you have flawless skin, a less-is-more approach, or maybe you're just too darn busy to spend twenty minutes pampering your skin before bed. All of those are perfectly good reasons. These are the products you should be using (there's an "optional" tag next to the ones that you can pass on if you'd like). That way you can sort of build your own nighttime routine. Do you want to use two products? Four? Eight? It's up to you.

- **Step 1: Cleanser/Makeup Remover**—This really shouldn't be optional for anyone. Think about all of the germs you've been in contact with all day, and all the times you've subconsciously touched your face. Now imagine all those germs spreading onto your pillowcase, clogging your pores, and causing breakouts. Also, if you wear makeup, cleanser or makeup remover is a *must*. In fact, if you're wearing makeup, I would recommend using both a makeup remover and cleanser . . . that eyeliner can be stubborn.
- **Step 2: Mask** (Optional)—A mask gives the best results when used after cleansing but before applying other products. Bonus points if you also exfoliate before using the mask. You'll get rid of all that dead skin for a deeper penetration of product. Plus, they also make masks for eyes, frown lines, and lips. Surely there's one out there for your needs.
- **Step 3: Toner** (Optional)—Toner is great if you're oily or acne prone. Plus, it can help get rid of any makeup or sunscreen remnants. My favorite thing about toner, though, is that it helps balance your skin's pH.
- **Step 4: Serum**—We already confirmed that your skin's permeability is enhanced at night. Serums are composed of small molecules that are designed to penetrate through the cell membrane. Meaning, nighttime is the best time to reap those benefits, whether it be for acne, wrinkles, hydration, etc.
- **Step 5: Moisturizer**—This is where the great night cream debate comes in. Whether you believe in them or not, use some kind of moisturizer that suits your skin needs. This one is also pretty important.
- **Step 6: Eye Cream** (Optional)—In all honesty, I do try to keep my skincare routine to a minimum, but I must say, I'm a huge fan of eye cream. Don't expect any overnight magic, but with consistent use it can help hydrate your undereye and

stave off aging. Plus, it's such a neglected area. Give it some extra love.

- **Step 7: Spot Treatment** (Optional)—If you have any blemishes, now's the time to dry those suckers out. It's also perfect for nighttime because you can go to sleep with paste dots on your face without having to worry about other people seeing you.
- **Step 8: Face Oil** (Optional)—Some people like to top off their evening routine with a facial oil for extra hydration. Don't worry about how dewy you might be. You're going to sleep, after all.

High-Maintenance Night Routine

If you prefer the full-on, royal-treatment, skin-as-soft-as-a-baby's-bottom approach, this section is for you. Naturally, I would assume you would want to do all of the steps outlined in the "low-maintenance" description, so I won't repeat those. Instead, here are some additional steps and products you can incorporate. You might not want to do all of these every day, but it could be good leading up to a special occasion—or if you've just had a long day at work dealing with passive-aggressive emails.

- **Cleansing Brushes**: Although many people think these devices are for exfoliation, they're actually more of a cleansing system. I'm sure you know about the craze with versions like Clarisonic and FOREO that hit the market a few years ago. Both are hand-held devices that use sonic technology to provide a deep cleanse. Clarisonic oscillates at a rate of 300 movements per second and has been said to remove six times more dirt, oil, and makeup than regular cleansing. The FOREO LUNA is made of bacteria-resistant silicone and moves at 8,000 pulsations per minute. Both are said to help with acne, wrinkles, and penetration of skincare topicals, but a lot of people get mixed results—hence their decline in recent years. Some people actually found that they were breaking out from using them, while others found the "exfoliation" to either be too irritating or not powerful enough. I wouldn't recommend using it on a daily basis, but I think it can be effective for the occasional deep clean.

- **Light Therapy Mask**: We already touched upon these a bit in the previous chapter, but some people really do swear by these and use them on a regular basis. Companies like Neutrogena have made them less expensive and more accessible. The LED lights are designed to help reduce inflammation and kill the bacteria associated with acne. Plus, it can also serve as a make-shift Darth Vader mask for Halloween.

- **Dermaroller**: We also touched upon this in the last chapter, but there are women who use this on a weekly/monthly basis. A dermaroller is a device that uses more than 500 stainless-steel needles to create micro injuries on your face. It tricks your body into producing more collagen and elastin to heal the wound and gradually fade wrinkles and acne scars. There is a wrong way to use it, though, so I would be careful to educate yourself on proper use before purchasing. You don't want a face full of scars.

- **Jade/Rose Quartz Roller**: If the dermaroller is too scary for you, might I introduce you to the jade roller? There are absolutely no needles so you don't have to worry about puncturing holes in your face. Tons of bloggers and celebrities swear by them, even though they look pretty unassuming. Jade rollers have actually been used since the seventeenth century in China and are said to remove toxins from the skin, smooth wrinkles, ease headaches, brighten the skin, calm inflammation, depuff eyes, etc. There are plenty of skeptics out there, but I say there's no harm in using one. If nothing else, it's super relaxing and makes a pretty decoration for your bathroom.

- **Face Steamer**: Facial steamers are rarely talked about, but there has been a surge of at-home devices on the market as of late. A facial steamer allows for deeper penetration of product, adds moisture back into the skin, and helps clear blackheads. Just make sure your skin is clean and don't go overboard by using it every day. It'll feel like your own at-home facial.

- **Facial Toner**: Facial toning devices like NuFace use electricity (in tiny amounts, of course) to shock your face. This stimulates facial muscles and causes them to contract, while enhancing the body's ability to make collagen and elastin, repair cells, and stimulate circulation. It's designed to mimic the effects of a facelift and can be used several times a week to prevent wrinkles.

- **Massage**: If facial toners are too intense for you (or the other devices break the bank) try a simple face massage using your own hands. There are tons of YouTube tutorials on how to do it correctly but it usually involves face oil, big circular motions, and lymph drainage. It's relaxing and can help boost your immune system and prevent wrinkles.

- **Exfoliation**: Facial exfoliation can happen in a variety of ways: cleansing brushes, peels, pore extraction, sugar polishes, etc. Find the best option that works for you and don't exfoliate more than once or twice a week. You want it to be effective without causing irritation.

CHAPTER 4

Whole Body

J'm sure I don't need to tell you this, but your body is not just your face. You knew that, right? I'm sure you've seen your other appendages at some point—hopefully moisturized them once or twice?

You've probably heard a lot of people say "it's okay to use face products for the rest of your body, but it's not okay to use body products for your face." Well, it's true. That's because your face and body have different needs when it comes to things like moisturizers. Your face tends to be a lot more sensitive and therefore requires more sensitive formulations. Your body, on the other hand, can handle thicker formulas like creams and body butter, especially on some of those trickier spots—anyone else have eternally dry elbows? Body moisturizers also aren't designed for areas with thinner skin, like around the eyes. There are different types of moisturizers you can use on your body—both by ingredients and consistency. We'll also navigate the difference between soaps and bodywashes, the history of body oil, and the age-old question that has our country divided: which is better, baths or showers?

Moisturizers

Are you sick of hearing about moisturizers yet? No? Me neither. In case you didn't know, moisturizers don't actually add moisture to the skin. Instead, they attract and secure existing water. First, let's break them down by ingredients and then by consistency to determine which is the best for your skin type. We have a lot to cover, so let's dive in. Moisturizers can generally be categorized by four types:

Humectants are ingredients that absorb moisture from the air and draw water up from deep layers of the skin to keep the skin hydrated. For this reason, they work best in humid climates where they have a steady supply of moisture in the air. Overall, humectants work well for all skin types (including sensitive skin because they're free of heavier oils), but are especially effective for those with dry skin. Ironically, they don't work so well for chronically dehydrated skin. That's because they can actually accelerate moisture loss from the deeper layers of skin. Once water reaches the outer layer of skin, it evaporates into the air—making it counterintuitive. That's why humectants are usually paired with occlusives (we'll get to that later). Most moisturizers are already formulated taking this into account, though, so there's no need to worry. Some examples of humectants include: glycerin (the most popular), alpha hydroxy acids (AHAs), sorbitol, urea, and everyone's favorite, hyaluronic acid (it can actually hold 1,000 times its weight in water).

Emollients are derived from plants and minerals that contain lipids, which naturally make up the structure of your skin. They're usually oil-based, but can be water-based. They fill in gaps between skin cells that are missing lipids to make your skin softer and smoother. A subclass of emollients, also known as "rejuvenators," provide essential proteins like collagen, elastin, and keratin. These types of proteins are too large to penetrate the skin but fill spaces on the outermost layer and improve elasticity. Other common examples of emollients include: colloidal oatmeal and shea butter. Emollients are best for extremely dry or mature skin because they not only hydrate, but can help reduce the appearance of wrinkles.

Occlusives form a hydrophobic (water-repellent) film to reduce water loss from the skin. Essentially, they create a protective seal over your skin so that you can't lose moisture. They're typically known as being the heaviest of moisturizers and will even feel kind of greasy when applied to the skin. That's why they're usually recommended for the body and not so much for the face. In fact, some people say that they're too effective. Not only do they trap water, but they also trap anything else that's on your face, meaning they can definitely trigger breakouts. As a result, occlusives are best for mature, dehydrated skin in an environment that's free of humidity. Some examples include: carnauba wax, lanolin, mineral oils, olive oil, petrolatum, and silicone. All-natural oils like rose hip, avocado, and hazelnut are also considered occlusives. Even though they're not great for sensitive skin, they can actually do wonders for skin issues like eczema—an issue I'm very familiar with, unfortunately.

Ceramides aren't technically moisturizers, but are super similar and usually grouped in this category. They're naturally found in the skin and are thought of as the "glue" holding the structure of your skin together. They make up about half of your skin's natural moisture barrier and also help regulate your cell's activity. Basically, damaged ceramide levels often lead to dry, damaged skin. Ceramides work best for normal and combination skin types, but they're also great for eczema (which is why a lot of people use CeraVe for Ceramides). If you have eczema, chances are that your ceramide levels are lower than they're supposed to be. Fun fact: synthetic and plant-derived ceramides are identical to the ones found in your skin.

Okay, so now let's break them down by consistency. So many of us use terms like "lotion," "cream," and "gel" interchangeably, but there are actually differences between all of them that are agreed upon in the skincare industry. It's true that all of these products are a mixture of lipid and water, but they vary in ratio. Water alone is a weak moisturizer because it evaporates quickly and doesn't protect your skin very well. Straight up lipids/oils tend to be too thick and gooey, which can clog your pores and trap bacteria. That's why most moisturizers fall somewhere in the middle of the spectrum:

Lotions are the lightest out of the three main types of moisturizers because water is their main ingredient—making them ideal for oily skin. Since their lipid content is lower, they tend to have a thinner consistency. Lotions are easy to spread, absorb quickly, and feel oh-so-light on the skin. But, they usually need to be applied more frequently to maintain proper hydration. Even if you have dry skin, lotions are great during the summer months when the air is hot and humid. Okay, now for the bad news. Lotions have the most added ingredients because they have such a high water content. Basically, the more water that's in a product, the more likely bacteria is to grow. To combat this, brands tend to add preservatives like parabens and benzyl alcohol. Since those preservatives tend to smell bad, they then add fragrance to mask the scent. Ugh! Not good for sensitive skin types. It's the reason why a lot of people choose to use lotion on the body and not the face. If your skin burns after applying a lotion, it's not a good kind of burn. It means that lotion probably isn't for you.

Creams are the middle ground between lotions (the lightest) and ointments (the heaviest). Basically, they're typically formulated with half water and half oil. A cream helps moisturize dry skin without feeling too heavy or greasy, making it ideal for those with normal to dry skin. A lot of people will switch from a lotion to a cream during the winter or dry months for extra hydration. Others prefer only to use creams at night because they feel they're too greasy or heavy for daytime. Creams are also ideal for those stubborn areas that we'll talk about later (elbows, feet, knees, etc.).

Ointments have the highest lipid ratio and therefore have the greatest moisturizing effect. This also tends to make them feel sticky and greasy.

Ointments are usually about 80 percent lipid and 20 percent water, but petroleum jelly (like Vaseline), is actually 100 percent lipid and no water. Ointments form a barrier that seals moisture into the skin, making them ideal for dry and itchy skin. They can also help relieve chapped skin/lips during the cold winter months. Like creams, ointments are also great for eczema. Okay, I'm done talking about eczema for a while. But if you suffer from it, you know the irritation is real.

Gels aren't technically a part of the holy trilogy of moisturizers, but are sometimes grouped in the same category. Gels are usually a mixture of water, lipid, and alcohol. They tend to feel cool and refreshing on the skin because they evaporate quickly after applying. Gels tend to feel even lighter and less greasy than lotions.

Body butters are somewhere in between cream and ointment. They're thick and creamy but also contain fatty oils (shea, coconut, cocoa butter, argan, olive, almond, etc.) to help your skin stay moisturized for a long time. Body butter works best on the driest areas of your body, which include those stubborn areas we keep mentioning. If you don't like the residue they leave, apply them at night so they have time to soak into your skin.

Soaps and Bodywash

This chapter is going to feel a bit competitive. First, we weighed the pros and cons of different moisturizers, later we'll have a bath vs. shower duel, and now we're going to let soap and bodywash fight it out. I'm sure if you're reading this, you have an opinion on which you prefer.

Soap, by definition, is a long chain of fatty acid alkali salt that usually has a pH between nine and ten. Since the body's natural pH is between five and six, bar cleansers tend to be harsh on the skin. They often remove lipids and proteins found on the skin's surface that help it retain

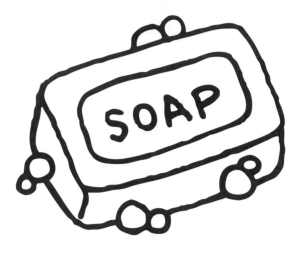

moisture. This often allows water to evaporate out of the skin and irritants to come in. That's because bar soaps are designed to make you feel squeaky-clean and are therefore made with lye or other ingredients that take away oil—often too much oil.

Most dermatologists recommend staying away from traditional bar cleansers for this reason, but newer formulations are better at remedying these issues. Artisanal bars, for example, are usually made with essential oils and shea butter, which is all you really need to get rid of dirt and bacteria. Translucent bar soaps are made with glycerin (a humectant that we just discussed which is known to draw moisture) to counteract the drying effect of soap. Superfatted soaps are formulated with lipids (which we *also* just discussed) to create a protective film over your skin. Combination bars combine surfactants (the harsh stuff) with natural oils to help nourish the skin. Syndet bars are formulated with synthetic surfactants and detergent (known for being softer on the skin). Meanwhile, some dermatologists just recommend using something like Dove (no, this is not #sponsored), because it's formulated with a mix of mild cleansers and essential nutrients.

Generally speaking, bar cleansers are more drying than body-wash because they contain chemicals like sodium hydroxide, whereas bodywashes are usually formulated with extra moisture to replace what the cleanser strips away. But some experts don't think the job of soap should be to moisturize; that's something that can be dealt with after your shower. In terms of getting clean, though, bar soap is just as effective as bodywash—even after your most intense workout.

However, there is a debate about whether bar soaps can create bacteria on its surface, especially if it's left in a moist environment. Generally, you should replace your soap once a month and try not to share it with any roommates. But studies have shown that there's actually little risk in sharing soap—cue the line from *Friends* where Chandler says, "Soap is soap, it's self-cleaning" and Joey says, "All right, well, next time you take a shower, think about the last thing I wash and the first thing you wash." At the end of the day, your skin is the first defense against bad things from the outside world, so it's important to keep it clean.

Like bar soap, **bodywash** is a cleanser that uses surfactants to cleanse the skin. The main difference is really their consistency—bodywash tends to be thinner. As we know, bodywashes tend to be more hydrating than bar soaps because they usually contain emollients. Newer formulations especially not only whisk away dirt, but actually deposit rich moisturizers that stick to the skin. In addition to essential oils, some even contain ceramides (we already know that those actually replenish your skin's surface). Another super important thing to note is that bodywash tends to have a neutral pH,

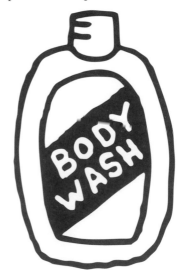

which is much closer to your skin's natural state. These are all great reasons why many people prefer bodywash over bar soap.

It's not always rainbows and butterflies though—some bodywashes do contain harsh surfactants like sodium laureate sulfate, which is similar to a compound found in dish soap that strips the skin of its natural oils. They also tend to have artificial fragrances, which can irritate the skin. When you use a bodywash, you also tend to use a loofah or washcloth, which can be breeding grounds for mold and bacteria. So that's something else to be mindful of.

Overall, I think most people these days have hopped on the bodywash bandwagon. It's usually less harsh, cleaner, and better for travel. There are some people who are die-hard bar soap users, though, and that's okay. Just make sure to check the ingredients for antibacterial agents like triclosan and triclocarbon that are known to strip away the good bacteria on skin—it can actually make you more vulnerable to bad bacteria and destroy your gut bacteria. Oh, and always moisturize.

Body Oil through the Years

Ah, body oils. Over the past few decades, there has been a bit of a fear instilled in us when it comes to using them: it will make you oily, it's terrible for acne, etc. But the movement toward clean beauty has rebirthed the love and importance of body oils. Skincare products you use seep into your skin, bloodstream, and even organs, so you want to use the purest substances, right? So, what exactly are essential oils? Essential oils are the aromatic oils extracted from parts of the plant, which include: flowers, leaves, seeds, roots, stems, bark, and wood. I've heard so many positive stories about the before-and-after effects of incorporating them into your routine, but the truth is, it isn't a new concept—humans have been using them for thousands of years. Carrier oils are vegetable oils that come from the seed, nut, or kernel of a plant. Carrier oils dilute the potency of essential oils (which can sometimes be too abrasive for the skin/body) and literally "carry" them into the skin.

Some examples of carrier oils include coconut, jojoba, avocado, rose hip, and sea buckthorn oils.

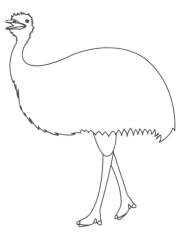

Aborigines living in Australia are presumably the first to start using oil—emu oil, to be exact—which they used as a moisturizer for more than 40,000 years. Woah. The oil is made from the pad fat on the emu's back and is known to treat skin conditions and arthritis as well.

Ancient Egyptians have been using oils as early as 4500 B.C.E. They became known for their knowledge of cosmetology and ointments— the most famous of their mixtures being "Kyphi," which was used as incense, perfume, and medicine. Archaeologists have also determined from burial sites and hieroglyphics that they used plant-based oils on the skin: castor, olive, and sesame (the latter two being Cleopatra's favorites). Fenugreek and moringa oils were used for sun and sand damage because they have antioxidants and boost circulation.

Oils were actually so valuable in Ancient Egypt that they were even used as a form of payment. That's because everyone from royalty to laborers used oils. In the twelfth century B.C.E, workers even went on strike because they complained they had no ointment and depended on the oils to ease their sore muscles after a long day of construction. At the height of Egypt's power, though, only members of the nobility were allowed to use oils because they were regarded as being divine. Fragrances were even dedicated to deities and pharaohs so that they could have their own special blend.

Oils were discovered in Egyptian graves that consisted of flowers and goose grease. Elite women were specifically known to lather themselves in these oils—scenes show they used to wear cones on their heads with oils on top of their wigs so that the scent released evenly throughout the day. They were also transported to the tombs of important people—oils were often kept in pottery jars. As Egyptians moved toward the Nile, they brought their love of fragrance with them.

Essential oils were used in the embalming process for mummification. Calcite pots with scented oils still held a faint smell when King Tutankhamen's tomb was opened 3,000 years later. Egyptians quickly became known for incredibly potent mixtures.

As in the modern day, ancient Egyptians also used them for beauty and skincare treatments. The first beauty spa ever was likely one owned by Cleopatra at En Gedi. Unfortunately, the book with her recorded recipes is long lost. How cool would it have been to use the exact same treatments as Cleopatra?

Unfortunately, the oils weren't always beneficial when it came to beauty. Female pharaoh Hatshepsut suffered from a severe dermatological condition and likely caused her own premature death by slathering herself with a mixture of palm oil, nutmeg oil, and benzopyrene (a tar that's very carcinogenic). Not a great sell for moisturizer, eh?

The Romans actually imported most of their oils from Egypt—the formulation process was a bit too messy for them. Romans literally bathed in oils and fragrance. Roman philosopher Pliny the Elder talked about the benefits of almond and castor oil when it comes to wrinkles, dark spots, and complexion. Dominican monks specifically would mix up avocado and macadamia oils to use as a nourishing night cream—fun fact: they're still sold today.

The Greeks bathed in essential oils and copied the Egyptians' use of oils somewhere between 400–500 B.C.E In Athens, *unguentarii* shops would sell marjoram, lily, thyme, sage, anise, rose, and iris infused with oil and beeswax. They would package them in small decorative pots, as they still do today. During those times, the shopkeepers were thought of as doctors, so their products were mostly used for medicinal purposes. Greeks would also use fragrance to enhance their sensuality—assigning a different scent for each part of the body. Oils were also used for massaging tight muscles, especially for athletes.

The Greeks are mainly known for their extensive oil use when it comes to medicinal purposes. Hippocrates, known as the "Father of Medicine," wrote about the effects of hundreds of plants and used his extensive knowledge for Ayurvedic techniques. He believed that having an oil bath and massage everyday was the way to good health. Galen, another Greek physician, was also known for his vast knowledge of plants and medicine. He began as a surgeon for gladiators (it is said that no gladiator died of a wound under his care) and was eventually hired as the personal physical to the Roman emperor. He's also credited with making cream a mass-marketed skincare product. "Galen's Wax" was a blend of olive oil, beeswax, and rosewater and is considered to be the first cold cream—it's actually what inspired modern-day formulas like Pond's and Nivea.

India is mostly known for its "Ayur Veda" approach, which we briefly touched upon with Hippocrates. Ayur Veda is a form of traditional Indian medicine that has a 3,000-year-old history of utilizing over 700 essential oils; the oils were believed to balance body temperature, temperament, and digestion. During the bubonic plague pandemic, it was even successfully used to replace antibiotics. A sesame oil blend was also a part of the daily bathing ritual. Generally speaking, women would

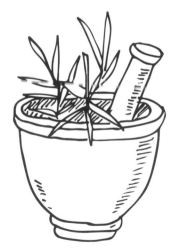

adorn themselves with certain oils in certain parts of the body, similar to the Greeks.

In **China**, the use of oils was first documented somewhere between 2697–2597 B.C.E. during the reign of Huang Ti. His renowned book, *The Yellow Emperor's Book of Internal Medicine,* includes uses for several aromatics and is still considered useful in Eastern medicine today.

In **Persia**, physician Ali-Ibn Sana (who lived from 980–1037 A.D.) wrote books on the healing benefits of 800 plants. He's also credited for being the first person to distill essential oils, and his methods are still used today.

Oils didn't reach **Europe** until the Crusades. Knights and their armies passed on knowledge that they learned about plants and distillation from the Middle East and even began carrying perfume on them. During the bubonic plague pandemic of the fourteenth century, frankincense and pine were burned in the street to ward off evil spirits. French chemist René-Maurice Gattefossé coined the term "aromatherapie" in 1928 while investigating the medicinal properties of essential oils. He actually discovered the amazing healing properties of lavender when an explosion happened at his lab. One of his hands was badly burned, so he ran it under lavender. He was surprised when his hand healed with no infections or scars.

Over the last two hundred years, a lot has changed. In eighteenth-century America, hog lard was used as a skin moisturizer—yikes. Mineral oils also became popular in the late nineteenth century with the creation of petroleum cream, jellies, and baby oils. They eventually dipped in popularity because they were said to clog pores and cause cancer, but that has since been proven wrong. In 1846, Pond's Creams were infused with witch hazel to heal burns. In recent years, essential oils have taken the high-end beauty industry by storm. In 2007, Josie Maran brought argan oil from Morocco, which, although technically a carrier oil, still helped spawn the hair and skincare trend almost everyone has tried.

In summation, go treat yourself to a luxury body oil or stop off at Whole Foods on your way home from work to pick up an essential oil infusion—you're already going there to get your avocados and Larabars anyway. Your body will thank you later.

Baths vs. Showers

Sure, most of us take showers on a daily basis, but when it comes to baths, you either love them or hate them. We already have enough divide in this country with our current political climate, so let's settle this one once and for all! Well, kind of. Once again, there are pros and cons to each one.

Okay, let's address one of the biggest concerns with **baths** first: you're not soaking in filth. Dirt tends to move away from the skin and body before getting diluted in the water. But, if you're really that concerned, you could always cleanse yourself in the shower and then bathe afterward. Baths are also great for relaxation and can even help lower cortisone levels, which helps delay aging and reduce acne. Soaking in the tub for just twenty minutes can help regulate blood pressure and improve circulation in the same way exercise does—so you can basically skip your 6:00 a.m. HIIT class. Elevating your body temperature can also boost your body's ability to fight infection and enhance oxygen flow throughout your respiratory system. There's even a term for

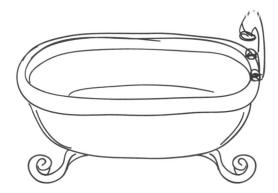

the treatment of disease through bathing called balneotherapy—just another reason to spend the day at the spa if you ask me.

In terms of skincare, baths have an advantage over showers in that you can add ingredients to the water. For sore muscles, use Epsom salt and for eczema, sunburn, inflammation, etc. add colloidal oatmeal, whole milk, and honey. You can even try those essential oils we talked about earlier. Just don't use anything that bubbles—I know, I know, no fun. But it's usually a sign that they contain detergents, which strips your skin of natural oils and moisture. This is usually true of beloved bath bombs also.

Baths are great so long as you don't spend too much time in there— it's not good for your skin to dehydrate it—and be sure to moisturize after.

Showers: ol' reliable. Showers may not be quite as relaxing as baths, but I find them to be rather relaxing. If you exercise regularly or wear a lot of makeup, showers are the way to go—this would be a case where you might be somewhat bathing in "filth." Showers are also better when washing your hair. It's obviously more difficult to rinse in a bath, plus sitting in shampoo will likely strip your skin of its natural oils. Like baths, just be sure not to take super-long showers because that can also dry out your skin.

Generally speaking, most experts agree that neither one is better than the other because each have good and less favorable qualities. It's rather a choice of personal preference.

Before we leave this topic entirely, let's figure out what pruning is. Why on earth do my fingers get wrinkly when I've been submerged in water too long? Is it worse to take a bath because of this reason? No, go ahead and take your bath. Pruning is believed to improve our grip while under water. After about five minutes under water, the sympathetic nervous system signals for constriction of the blood vessels on the skin on your fingers, palms, toes, and soles shrivel so that we can easily pick up wet or submerged objects. Evolution is pretty amazing. They work kind of like tire treads to allow us to pick up that bar of soap you just dropped . . . or bodywash? Experts don't know why we don't just have grip-like fingers all the time, but I'd like to think it's because we get to transform like superheroes.

Foot Care

Foot care is a complicated and somewhat embarrassing topic. I can honestly say I've had virtually every issue when it comes to feet, but for the sake of your sanity, I'll spare you the details. Some people only require a simple washing and moisturizing, while others need exfoliation, sweat protection, and treatments. If you're lucky enough to have daily pedicures, then congratulations: you've made it in life. You likely have a personal chef and diamond curtains as well. If you're a regular person and have to tend to your own feet on a daily basis, here's what you need to know:

To cleanse, soak your feet in a bath for ten to fifteen minutes to soften the skin. You can even add black tea to prevent the risk of athlete's foot. Some experts insist you don't even need to soak your feet because it will simply dehydrate them. Instead, you can apply a sugar scrub directly to the dry skin and remove it with a damp towel.

Most experts would recommend exfoliating at least once a week (which I definitely don't do . . . whoops). You can do this by keeping a pumice stone in your shower, using a foot scrub, or using a foot file while your heels are still damp—this will help get rid of calluses and dry skin. If you want to bring in the big guns, you can try a chemical peel. Yes, I know, you thought they were only for your face, but they're not. Amlactin Foot Cream Therapy uses AHAs so that literal flakes of skin fall off your heels after a few days of use. If you're really into it, you can also try Baby Foot. If you thought the flakes were big for Amlactin, you should see the ones that come off after using this. Baby Foot promises to get rid of the roughest calluses to reveal smooth skin. In less than a week, you'll start to shed your foot cocoon to reveal beautiful new butterfly feet.

Once you've exfoliated, it's time to moisturize. Your heels are especially prone to overuse so it's important to protect the skin with a lotion immediately after your shower. There are special creams prescribed for those tough areas like heels and elbows. I've seen many people recommend Glytone Ultra Softening Heel and Elbow Cream but you can also try Bliss softening socks, Lush Volcano Foot Mask, or anti-callus salve (once again, none of these are #sponsored). Don't forget about those toenails, though! Simply use a cuticle cream, petroleum jelly, or vitamin E oil.

Speaking of toes, you didn't think I'd forget about nail care, did you? Other than tweezers and a nail file, the most important tip I can give you is this: don't wear nail polish all the time. Your nails need a break to breathe in order to grow and prevent discoloration.

If you made it this far, I'm proud of you. I wanted to see if you could handle the less-glamorous stuff. It's not all fun and games with beauty. Sometimes you have to use products that aren't fun. No glitter, no color, no fancy packaging. My last piece of footcare advice: if you're prone to sweat, you're also likely prone to athlete's foot and nail fungus. In terms of prevention, you can try deodorant (the same one you use for your armpits), foot powder, feet wipes, or foot spray. If you're in too deep and you're now solving the problem, there are tons of treatments out there for foot and nail fungus relief. Whatever you do, don't neglect it. It'll only get worse over time.

CHAPTER 5

Sun Protection

If you're spending all this time, money, and energy to have beautiful skin, then I sure hope you're wearing sunscreen every day to ensure it *stays* beautiful . . . yes, *every day*. There's no use in those fancy night creams and treatments if you're just going to end up with wrinkles and sun spots anyway, right? If you're not wearing it every day, chances are you're misinformed: about UV rays, their presence, types of sunscreens, using it with makeup, etc. Sunscreen is super important for everyone—not just if you're pale, live somewhere tropical, or spend hours in the

sun on a daily basis. Science has some serious facts to back this up and unlike the previous chapter, most of this stuff is universally agreed upon by experts. In fact, contrary to popular belief, there are *no* positive effects of UV rays on the skin (unless someone has psoriasis or a skin disease that improves with UV therapy). If you're vitamin D deficient, you can take a supplement! UV rays also don't improve Seasonal Affective Disorder (SAD); it's broad spectrum light, which you can get from those boxes. So, there's no excuse why you shouldn't be wearing sunscreen.

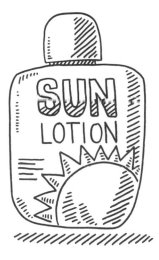

If I don't have you on board with daily sunscreen use yet, I guarantee I will by the end of this chapter. In fact, $20 says I will. We all want to look forty when we're sixty, right?

Sunscreen vs. SPF

Even though many people use "sunscreen" and "SPF" interchangeably, they're not actually the same thing. Sunscreen, by definition, contains ingredients that help absorb UV rays and convert the sun's radiation into heat energy, which reflects and scatters the rays so that they don't seep into the skin. SPF is an acronym that stands for "sun protection factor," which refers to the amount of time after application that you can spend in the sun without getting burned. For instance, an SPF of 30 would allow you to stay in the sun thirty times longer than if you were wearing no sunscreen. So basically, "sunscreen" refers to the physical protection from the sun whereas "SPF" is simply a unit of measure for it.

Types of Rays

Okay, if you don't already know the difference between rays, this is important because once you know, it might change your mind on the whole "wearing sunscreen daily" thing:

- **UVA:** Ultraviolet A rays, or "short waves," make up 95 percent of the rays that reach the Earth's surface. They penetrate your skin much more deeply than UVB rays, which is why they're responsible for damage that happens in the deeper layers of your skin—a.k.a. age-related signs like wrinkles and sun spots. Most importantly, they also cause skin cancer like melanoma. Even scarier, UVA damage is essentially irreversible, which means protection against it is super important. If you weren't already scared by their power, UVA rays can also penetrate glass and clouds—meaning the excuses "but I'm inside all day" or "it's cloudy outside" are no good.

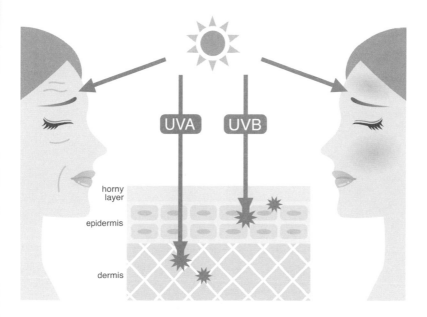

horny
layer

epidermis

dermis

- **UVB**: Ultraviolet B rays, or "short waves," make up the much smaller percent that reaches the Earth's surface and don't penetrate the skin as deeply as UVA rays. They're mainly responsible for redness and sunburns—so the more immediate, temporary, and superficial symptoms ("superficial" meaning on the surface . . . not someone who values beauty over brains. Although, if someone thinks less of you because of your accidental lobster skin then forget about them). UVB rays are most intense from the early spring to early fall and during the day's sunniest hours (10:00 a.m.–4:00 p.m.). Even though they do die down in the winter, they can still be reflected off snow and ice, which is why you get sunburn when skiing or even shoveling snow. Unlike UVA rays, though, they're less likely to penetrate glass and clouds.

- **HEVL**: High Energy Visible Light is infrared blue light that's emitted from your electronic devices (phones, tablets, computers, etc.) and penetrates even *deeper* than the sun's UV rays. It's believed to seriously increase the signs of aging, including delayed cell recovery and hyperpigmentation. There hasn't been enough research conducted yet, so no need to *completely* freak out, but I definitely think it's something to be mindful of over the coming years. Japan has already started factoring this in when making skincare products, and the United States has slowly started to follow suit. You can now find sunscreens that claim to protect from HEVL. But if you were looking for another excuse to stay off social media, this is it.

As you can see, UVA rays, which account for almost all of the Earth's rays, are visible all year round, while UVB rays are reduced but still present. You truly cannot escape them. This is why it's best to wear a broad-spectrum sunscreen year-round. Did I scare you into using it yet?

What If It's Not a Sunny Day?

Since we know that UVA rays are always present and UVB rays are only slightly lessened by clouds, you always need to wear sunscreen. Pretty much every dermatologist will tell you to wear it every season no matter what the weather forecast says or if you're spending the whole day inside. Even if you *only* spend twenty minutes a day outside (between taking out the trash, driving your car, running errands, etc.), that time will add up. UV damage is less about the amount of time spent outside in one sitting and rather about the accumulation of time spent outside. So, if you go all winter without wearing sunscreen, you're literally adding hundreds of hours a year to your sun damage.

Also, the winter can have its own intensity of UV damage. Did you know that snow and ice can reflect up to 90 percent of UV rays?

Meanwhile, the ozone, the Earth's natural sunshield, is actually the thinnest in the winter, making you more susceptible to harmful rays.

Another scary fact I bet you didn't know, UV damage is at its greatest when you're on a plane. You're closer to the sun so it makes sense, right? Radiation can also increase when flying over thick clouds or snowfields because they reflect up to 85 percent of the rays. Unfortunately, airplane windows don't really do a good enough job at protecting you, either. So, you should definitely be wearing sunscreen when on a plane and reapplying throughout the flight—if you're flying from New York to Australia, I'm sorry. You should maybe just bring a whole tube? Or whatever they'll let you get past airport security.

The good news is you can decrease your SPF in the cooler seasons if you'd like. Most experts recommend around SPF 45 or higher from May through September, but only SPF 30 from October through April. If you're like me, you'll just want to apply SPF 50 all year round just in case. Make sure it's always broad spectrum, seek shade during the sun's brightest hours, and check with a doctor to make sure none of your medication is phototoxic. You can also try clothing with UPF (Ultraviolet Protective Fabric), polarized sunglasses, and a hat. I'd rather be safe than sorry. They won't be laughing twenty years from now when you're wrinkle-free.

Physical vs. Chemical Sunscreen

Did you know there's a difference between sunscreens?

- **Physical**: contains active mineral ingredients, like titanium dioxide or zinc oxide, which sit on top of the skin to deflect and scatter damaging UV rays away from the skin. Think of the UV rays as a ball hitting the ground—it simply bounces back in the opposite direction. Physical sunscreens have recently gained popularity.

Pros:

- Naturally broad spectrum, offering protection from both UVA and UVB
- No wait time after application, protects from the sun ASAP
- Lasts longer in direct UV light
- Better for sensitive skin, less likely to cause irritation
- Better for those with "heat-activated" skin (rosacea and redness) since it deflects the heat from the sun away from the body
- Ideal for acne/blemish-prone skin since it's less likely to clog pores
- Longer shelf life

Cons:

- Can rub, sweat, and rinse off easily, meaning you'll need to reapply more frequently
- Can lend a white cast to the skin, making it less ideal for darker skin types
- Too chalky and thick to layer under makeup
- Must apply generous amounts since UV light can penetrate through the sunscreen molecules if applied unevenly

Chemical: contains organic compounds, such as oxybenzone, octinoxate, octisalate, and avobenzone, which create a chemical reaction to change UV rays into heat and then release it from the skin. Unlike the bouncing-ball analogy, chemical sunscreens actually absorb the UV rays into the top layers of the skin and just convert it to heat. Chances are, if you own a generic sunscreen, it's likely chemical.

<u>Pros:</u>
- Spreads more easily on the skin because it's thinner, making it ideal for daily use
- Less product is needed because there's no risk of space between the sunscreen molecules
- Easier to mix with other treatments, serums, and makeup

<u>Cons:</u>
- Can actually increase discoloration due to higher internal skin temperature
- Requires a wait time of at least ten minutes after application to create a protective film
- Increased chance of irritation and stinging, especially for sensitive skin types
- Protection it offers gets used up more quickly when in direct UV light, so you have to apply more frequently
- Increased chance of redness for rosacea-prone skin types because it converts the UV rays to heat
- Can damage oceans and coral reefs—save the planet!
- Can clog pores, especially for oily skin types
- Can sting if it gets into your eyes

Neither one is better or worse than the other per se. It all depends on personal preference. Some experts do believe that physical sunscreen might be better at blocking UVA rays, but that's not a universally accepted belief.

I'm acne-prone so I tend to prefer physical sunscreens to prevent breakouts, but chemical sunscreens are better if I'm wearing makeup that day. On the other hand, if I know it's sweltering or I'm going to be exercising outside, chemical is usually the way to go because I know I won't have white beads of sweat dripping down my face. No matter which one you choose, it's better than wearing none!

Antioxidants

Some experts believe that even more important than the SPF number on a sunscreen bottle is its ingredients. Even while wearing sunscreen, some UV rays can still penetrate the skin and cause oxidation or "free radical damage." Wearing a sunscreen formulated with antioxidants will prevent that. In fact, sunscreens should always include hydrators, anti-inflammatory properties, and antioxidants—together, they'll help repair the skin's barrier to protect itself from the sun, bacteria, and pollution. If your sunscreen doesn't have antioxidants, you can layer it with a serum that has green tea polyphenols, vitamin C and E.

How Much Sunscreen/What SPF Should I Be Using?

In terms of sunscreen, the FDA insists that when it comes to your face and neck, you should be using ¼ teaspoon or 2.0 mg/cm2 to get the right amount of protection. It'll usually look like a nickel-sized amount. Most of us don't use as much as we should be, so you can always try measuring it out with a baking utensil to get a feel for it first.

In terms of SPF, the higher number, the more coverage, the better. There are rumors going around that anything above SPF 50 is unnecessary and ineffective—the FDA even put a limit on marketing anything above SPF 50—but most experts would disagree. The only thing you want to be careful about is not getting an inflated ego. Some people think that using SPF 50 means they don't need to reapply, but they're wrong. You still need to reapply every eighty minutes, at least. If you do happen to think SPF 50 is excessive, you're likely good with anything above SPF 30 in the summer. But if you have especially sensitive skin or aren't getting desirable results, take it up a notch.

Reapplication

Reapplication is super important. Reapplication has nothing to do with the "breaking down of ingredients" but instead has to do with sunscreen washing off through natural perspiration that happens throughout the day–it evaporates fast so that it doesn't accumulate on your skin which is why you usually don't feel it. You don't necessarily need to be exercising or swimming (although you should definitely be reapplying after you do both of those) for it to come off.

Generally, you should apply every eighty to 120 minutes, especially if you're sitting out in the sun. If you're inside most of the day, you can usually get away with just a morning application—so long as you apply enough and don't plan on getting happy-hour drinks outside after work.

Also, there's no such thing as waterproof sunscreen. Only water-resistant. So be sure to reapply after swimming, exercising, running through sprinklers (ah, the good old days), etc.

Sunscreen in Makeup and Skincare

A lot of skincare and makeup products these days are formulated with SPF protection. You're probably wondering, *is that enough?* It depends who you ask. Some experts might say it's okay to get your Sunscreen solely from makeup, but most agree it's best to wear a layer of sunscreen underneath it all.

A study presented at the British Association of Dermatologists annual meeting found that the sunscreen in our moisturizers isn't offering us enough UV protection. The results proved that moisturizers with sunscreen provide less protection than standard sunscreens with equal sunscreen strength. So basically, that sunscreen 15 in your favorite foundation is less effective than the sunscreen 15 in your Coppertone. Researchers used a special camera that captures UV light in order to look at the way that participants applied regular and moisturizer sunscreen. When an area is sufficiently covered with sunscreen, it appears black under the UV light. When they looked at the pictures of the people who applied moisturizer with sunscreen, their faces were much lighter, which implies that sunscreen absorption was less effective and successful. That's not to say you shouldn't buy skincare products with sunscreen in it, it just means it's not enough.

Therefore, although you can find many skincare and makeup products with sunscreen in them (foundations, concealers, moisturizers, serums, primers, CC creams, BB creams, setting powders, etc.) don't rely on those products as your only source of sun protection.

Sunscreen and Acne

As someone who struggles with acne, I can relate to the problem of not wanting to wear sunscreen for fear that I'll break out. I wear it anyways, but some days if I know I'm not leaving my house, I won't wear it. If you think you have problems with acne now, wait until the problems you'll get later from wearing no sunscreen. You're essentially trading in red blemishes for brown spots and wrinkles.

There are tons of oil-free sunscreens out there that protect your skin without clogging your pores. Also, remember we talked about the physical sunscreens before? They're better for acne-prone skin since they are composed of minerals and help keep the skin cooler. Also, if you're using Accutane or retinol to help with acne, they can actually make your skin even more sensitive to the sun.

One common concern with people who are acne-prone is reapplying throughout the day. It's one thing if you're applying first thing in the morning and your skin is freshly washed. But if you're reapplying later in the day, wouldn't you just be rubbing dirt and oil into your skin? What if I'm already wearing makeup? I can't take off all my makeup just to reapply my sunscreen and then *reapply* my makeup. There may not be one obvious answer—I simply choose not to wear makeup most days. However, one solution may be to mix a powder formulated with SPF along with a makeup powder that gives you a smooth finish and slight glow. When mixed together, they'll help protect your skin while ensuring it appears blemish-free and youthful.

Expiration Dates

All this talk about sunscreen but nothing about when you should throw yours away. I'm sure most of us are guilty of this: every spring I find myself rummaging through last year's beach bag for a sunscreen with a high SPF. No? Just me?

Most sunscreens list an expiration date but, the general rule of thumb is that they expire three years after purchase. However, this isn't always the case. One of the major problems with sunscreen is that most people are unintentionally destroying theirs; they let it sit at the bottom of their beach bag while baking in the sun all day. This is actually really bad (but realistically, super hard to prevent, right? I mean, you want me to reapply every eighty minutes and if I'm sitting on the beach, how can I trek back to an air-conditioned house every time to make sure my sunscreen stays safe for use?) Anyways, keeping sunscreen in the heat and light will cause it to break down faster—it becomes less effective, less stable, and less reliable. Anything above seventy-seven degrees Fahrenheit will usually degrade it.

As a general rule of thumb, throw it away if you notice the oil and product start to separate—I'm ashamed to say I haven't always done this—or if the sunscreen starts to turn yellow, grow moldy, or you notice it isn't effective in protecting your skin. I usually try to just buy a new sunscreen every April (SPF 50) and it usually lasts me until October—I'm pale and a baby about the heat so I don't spend too much time at the beach. I usually just need to cover my face, neck, and arms around that time. But if you're applying sunscreen every day, you shouldn't have to worry too much about weather a sunscreen is expired because you'll run out long before the expiration date. Plus, you don't want to waste a perfectly good sunscreen.

If the damage has already been done, it's never too late to start wearing SPF. Sure, there *are* treatments out there to help reverse the signs of sun damage, but it won't be easy to get rid of altogether. How can you not wear it every day now?

I think I earned my $20.

CHAPTER 6

Reading the Labels

Trying to make sense of a skincare label is like trying to make sense of a Shakespearean play—you kind of recognize some words and understand the general gist of what it's trying to say, but at the end of the day it's still a foreign language—does anyone else find Old English to be equally as confusing as scientific nomenclature? Sure, it's significant and should not be overlooked, but sometimes it's easier to use CliffsNotes to find out the important stuff: does it have parabens? Is it cruelty-free? What's in a name? A rose by any name would smell as sweet. Okay, the last one is a *Romeo and Juliet* quote, but offers sound advice for analyzing ingredients.

Knowing how to read a skincare label is important. Remember, the products we apply onto our skin seep into our bloodstream. You want to make sure you're not putting anything toxic into your body. Perhaps you also care a great deal about potency, animal cruelty, or the mysterious world of package symbols. There's also a lot of confusion with ambiguous terms like "natural," "organic," and "synthetic." Don't make assumptions. The FDA is very lax with their regulations when it comes to makeup and skincare, which means you're going to have to do research on your own. Luckily, I've taken away some of that burden. Just remember, "all that glitters is not gold."

What to Look for on a Skincare Label

This might seem like common sense, but ingredients on skincare labels are listed in the order of their concentrations—so if a face cream is 30 percent water and 20 percent glycerin, the water is listed first. There is an important exception to this rule, though: ingredients that are less than 1 percent of the formula (as well as colorants, fragrances, and preservatives) can be listed in any order among themselves. Naturally, the manufacturer is going to choose the more desirable ingredients to go first. This can obviously be misleading. Although the first five ingredients are typically the bulk of the formula, it doesn't mean that the lower percentage ingredients can't make an impact. In fact, ingredients like collagen-boosting peptides are extremely effective at low levels. Similarly, retinol and vitamin C can become painful or irritating to the skin if used at high percentages. These two examples might sound like pleasant surprises, but it can also be for the worse.

Another important caveat to note is that fragrances don't have to be listed at all. Instead, they're allowed to be listed under the guise of "parfum" or "aroma." This sounds sexy and French, I know, but fragrance is actually a bad thing—we'll get to that later. Once again, there's an exception to this rule. There are twenty-six fragrance compounds that do have to be listed if used due to the fact that they commonly cause allergic reactions—this seems so dumb, right? Why even use it!? We'll get to that later, too.

ACTIVE VS. INACTIVE INGREDIENTS:
Active ingredients are ones that are approved by the United States Food and Drug Administration (FDA) to perform a specific function for a certain condition. For example, titanium oxide is approved for sun protection, benzoyl peroxide for acne, and hydroquinone for skin lightening. On the label, they'll be listed with their percentages, a brief

description, and how it should be applied. Inactive ingredients aren't actually "inactive"—why would the brand waste their time including it? Inactive ingredients are simply ones that provide support or benefits to the formula. For instance, an acne-treating product might not say "acne" on the label, but it doesn't mean it won't treat it, and it might even contain salicylic acid. That's because the FDA actually regulates the word "acne" and "blemish" to include specific ingredients and percentages. Most brands just get around this by calling it "clarifying." Unfortunately, inactive ingredients also don't have to be proven safe prior to use. When in doubt, go for the one that lists the active ingredients.

INGREDIENTS WITH LONG NAMES:
I know, I know: you've been trained to think that all ingredients with long confusing names are bad. A lot of the time, this is true. But don't assume that just because it's unpronounceable that it's automatically a weapon of mass destruction. For example, acetyl hexapeptide-8 is a collagen-stimulating ingredient whose name describes its chemical structure. Ingredients with "edta" or "edds" in the name prevent the heavy metals in tap water from eating away at the beneficial ingredients in skincare. Similarly, emulsifiers (most of which have an "-eth" suffix) prevent the formula from separating in the bottle so that you get an even distribution of product with every application.

A lot of these long-named ingredients are also naturally derived . . . surprised? Here's a list of some examples:

- Tocopherol (vitamin E) protects the formula from expiring
- Xanthan gum thickens the product
- Cetyl alcohol and cetearyl alcohol have a moisturizing effect
- Citric acid regulates the pH levels and protects it from bacterial contamination
- Sorbitan olivate is an emulsifier that's made from a combination of sugar alcohol and olive oil

- Potassium sorbate is a preservative that's made from the salt of sorbic acid.

Some of these natural ingredients might even be plant-based, which is a good thing. That's because it's actually the Latin name of the botanical (which is always represented with two words representing Genus species). For example, lavender's scientific name is "*Lavandula angustifolia*" and we all know lavender has amazing properties that we wouldn't want to miss out on because of a common misconception. The reason that they're listed this way is because in the EU, cosmetic ingredients are required to be labeled using their INCI (International Nomenclature of Cosmetic Ingredients). To be honest, I'm not really sure of the reasoning other than that it prohibits any confusion as to whether it's a natural plant or false marketing. The bottom line is—do your research! You don't want to miss out on major results because you thought "*Melaleuca alternifolia*" was a deadly spell from Harry Potter.

INGREDIENTS YOU MAY FIND

I'm not going to delve into most of these because we've talked about them in previous chapters, but I thought I would list some of the more common ingredients you might find on skincare labels. They each serve a purpose which is why they were chosen for the formulation:

- **Water**: Usually the first ingredient in most skincare products. Sometimes aloe vera is used instead because it's packed full of nutrients.
- **Humectants**: Glycerin is by far the most common. We know that humectants keep your skin moisturized. Try to look for vegetable glycerin because it's plant-based.
- **Emulsifiers**: Help bind and thicken the formula. They can be natural or synthetic. Examples: E-wax, stearic acid, borax, soy wax, beeswax.

- **Proteins (Peptides)**: Some labels use the common name while others use the scientific nomenclature. This is an important ingredient.
- **Natural Botanicals**: We already talked about these Latin babes. They nourish your skin with essential vitamins and minerals, duh. There's a long, long list of wonderful botanicals but some common ones are: calendula, lavender, and green tea.
- **Preservatives**: Not a sexy word. Most are synthetic but some are actually natural like radish root, vitamin E, and grapefruit seed oil. They're usually used in small percentages, though (the 1 percent kind we talked about earlier).
- **Citric Acid**: used to regulate the pH of a formula.
- **Colorants**: give a formulation color to make them look aesthetically pleasing. Some are natural but many can actually be carcinogens, so be careful! They're also usually listed at the end, so don't get lazy by avoiding the last few ingredients listed.

BAD INGREDIENTS YOU MAY FIND

Sure, all ingredients serve a purpose, but the long-term effects may not be as beneficial as the short-term ones. Here are some you should definitely avoid (or at least be aware of):

- **Parabens**: let's start with the big guns. All skincare products that contain water also need some sort of preservative, and parabens are a synthetic option. Parabens are very common, but unfortunately also carcinogenic, irritating, and notorious for allergic reactions. They're known for disrupting our natural hormone cycles because they mimic estrogen and therefore trick our bodies into thinking we already have enough. They can also lead to DNA damage, increasing skin aging, and even cancer. You've probably seen tons of brands now stamping their labels with "paraben-free." If you're not sure where you might find them, they're usually in liquid-based products like shampoo, bodywash, lotion, foundation, etc. You can also check the ingredient list. Anything with the suffix "paraben" is indeed a paraben (methylparaben, butylparaben, ethylparaben, propylparaben, isobutylparaben). It's not always so straightforward, though. Phenoxyethanol, ethylhexylglycerin, hydroxybenzoic acid, and hydroxybenzoate are all versions of parabens that brands use to trick you into thinking there are no parabens.

- **Sulfates**: Sulfates are detergents and foaming agents that are usually found in cleaning products like face wash and shampoo. While many people think that they clean your skin, they actually just remove oil from it (yes, the good kind of oil, too) and lead to dehydrated skin. As you can imagine, this can lead to irritation and allergic reactions. They can also be contaminated with other ingredients that cause cancer and interfere with our body's natural functions. Similar to parabens, they're usually easy to spot. Look for ingredients that end in "sulfate" like lauryl sulfate, sodium laureth sulfate, ammonium lauryl sulfate, etc.

- **Phthalates**: are another group of chemicals that are found in hundreds of products. In the beauty industry, they can be found in lotions, fragrances, shampoos, and soaps because they help moisturize and soften the skin. Like the two other chemicals from before, they can lead to cancer, fertility issues, and organ damage. They can even cause birth defects, which is why they're banned in the EU. Look for labels that say "phthalates free" and also avoid anything that says DBP, DEHP, DEP, DMP, or fragrance. Anything with synthetic fragrances likely has phthalates.

- **Formaldehyde**: is that carcinogenic preservative that douses dead frogs—the one you used for dissection in your eighth-grade science class. So why on *earth* would you want that on your body? Not only does it cause skin irritation, but it also leads to cancer, asthma, and neurotoxicity. Formaldehyde is usually found in shampoo, bodywash, bubble bath, and hair dye. Some of these are a little harder to spot on ingredient lists. In addition to "formaldehyde," you should also steer clear of formaldehyde releasers like DD hydatoin, diazolidinyl urea, methanamin, and quarterium-15.

- **Silicones**: are controversial because they actually have some good benefits. Silicones form films that allegedly trap debris in your pores and prevent other ingredients from properly absorbing into your skin. They can also cause acne and dehydrated skin. Overall, it's considered a relatively safe chemical to use but some would rather err on the side of caution. Look for ingredients that end in "-cone," "-siloxane," or "-conol."

- **Coal-tar dyes**: are Polycyclic aromatic hydrocarbons (a type of chemical) that is found in coal, crude oil, and gasoline. Not surprisingly, they're carcinogenic and the FDA actually requires them to be put on the label if it contains 0.5 to 5 percent (the highest level allowed). They're mainly found in hair dye and anti-dandruff shampoos.

- **Ethanolamines (MEA/DEA/TEA)**: are chemicals that are used in cosmetics to make them creamy. They are known to cause allergic reactions, skin toxicity, hormone disruption, and birth defects. You can usually find them in hair dyes, mascara, foundation, fragrances, and sunscreens.

- **Fragrance**: You're probably so sick of hearing about the negative effects of fragrances. You're just trying to smell nice, I get it. The reality is that there is fragrance in virtually every cosmetic product. What's worse is that over 3,000 chemicals commonly used for fragrance have never been tested for toxicity. As we mentioned before, fragrance has a lot of loopholes when it comes to FDA regulations. But just because the government is lazy, it doesn't mean you should be, too. Fragrances are known to be hormone disrupters and cause allergic reactions. They also contain a lot of preservatives, dyes, and other bad stuff. I know it can be tempting, but try to steer clear of them. If you're looking for a pleasant aroma, try making your own blend of essential oils. That way you can truly have your own unique scent, too.

- **Petrolatum**: is a mineral oil jelly (think Vaseline, Aquaphor, etc.) that's used to lock in moisture. It's actually a deodorized form of kerosene . . . if that's any indication of how intense it is. It literally prevents the skin from breathing. Not going to lie, I love petrolatum. You'd have better luck getting me to stop sleeping than prying my Aquaphor out of my hands. Sadly, though, they are often contaminated with PAHs, which is why the EU considers them carcinogenic. They can be found in a variety of skincare items, though, including children's products. Double-check those ingredients if you're concerned.

- **BHA and BHT**: More confusing letters. BHA and BHT are synthetic antioxidants that are used as preservatives. As with almost every chemical we've mentioned, they are most likely carcinogenic, disrupt hormone function, and can cause reproductive issues. You'll usually find them in lipsticks and moisturizers.

- **Oxybenzone**: is often found in sunscreen because it absorbs ultraviolet light, but can also be found in nail polish, lip balm, fragrance, and hair products. It's linked to skin irritation, allergies, hormone disruption, and reproductive toxicity. As with many ingredients we've discussed, it's not restricted in the United States but is restricted up to 10 percent maximum concentration in the EU.

I think we've covered most of the major hazardous ingredients you should know about in skincare. It takes a while to feel comfortable reading a label, but if you're ever unsure about a product you're buy-ing, the Environmental Working Group has a "Skin Deep Guide to Cosmetics" online (and an app) where you can search over 80,000 products to check the breakdown of their ingredients. They even give them a safety rating from one to ten so that you know just how danger-ous the ingredients really are. You might be pretty disappointed to find out some of your favorite products are a solid "8".

SYMBOLS YOU MAY FIND

Symbols can be great: they're universal, take up less space, and save your brain from having to read—I know I'm not the only one who's become lazy from social media use. On the other hand, they can be confusing if you don't know what they mean or refuse to do your research. I won't cover *all* of the symbols—you guys know what the flame and recycling symbols mean, right? I'll just cover some of the ones that are more com-mon or indicate a certification:

- **Period-after-opening symbol**: A jar with a floating lid can often be found with a number and the letter *M*. This refers to the number of months the product is good for after opening. It's basically an expiration date. I guarantee at least a few of you will run to your medicine cabinet to check as soon as this section ends.
- **The Vegan Heart**: The Vegan Certified logo ensures that a product is formulated with vegan ingredients and is not tested on animals.
- **Leaping Bunny**: The leaping bunny logo ensures that the product is cruelty-free and has gone through a variety of rigor-ous testing and independent auditing. Make sure it's certified by Cruelty Free International, though. Some companies even go so far as to include their own version of a bunny just to make it seem cruelty-free.

- **Ecocert**: the Ecocert logo means the product has been inspected by one of the most prominent organizations in organic regulation. The organization is based in Europe and conducts inspections in over eighty countries. It's actually one of the largest certification companies in the world.
- **NSF**: Don't worry, it's not the same as NSFW. The NSF logo means that at least 70 percent of the ingredients are organic.
- **Lowercase e:** The "estimated sign" symbol ensures that the amount of product labeled is correct and you're not being ripped off. It's only found in products from the EU, though so if you strictly buy American, you likely won't come across it.

Ambiguous Terms

This might sound paranoid, but skincare brands use professional-sounding words and phrases to trick you. We've all seen it before. You'll pick up a box that'll say "all-natural," but what does that even mean? Is it certified? I barely know what any of these ingredients are! Sometimes, you probably don't even know you're being tricked. The FDA is very lax when it comes to regulations, and companies have figured out ways of getting around this. The terminology they use is specifically designed to trick you. If you don't believe me, here are some examples:

"Hypoallergenic" probably sounds pretty legit right? It must mean the company has done tons of testing on their product to ensure it won't cause an allergic reaction . . . nope. There are actually no FDA regulations that govern the use of terms like "hypoallergenic" on skincare products. A company can do extensive testing (or not) and still plaster it on their packaging if they want. The same goes for "**noncomedogenic**"—a term used for products that don't contain ingredients that clog up the pores. A product can also claim to be "oil-free" but still clog up your pores without containing oil. If you're acne prone, you can try to avoid this by looking for products with liquid and gel textures.

This one will surprise you: there are no FDA regulations for "**clinically proven**" or "**dermatologist-tested**," either. "Clinically proven" simply means the product went through some kind of test. It doesn't matter what kind, how many people were tested, what the results were, etc. The product can even contain harmful ingredients and still be labeled with "clinically tested." "Dermatologist-tested" usually means that a dermatologist has done a patch test to see if it caused an allergic reaction on the skin. It doesn't test to see if the product actually does any of the things it claims like reduce wrinkles, hydrate skin, etc. Another important thing to remember is that "dermatologist-tested" doesn't mean "dermatologist-endorsed." Just because they tested it doesn't mean that it's safe enough to use! What has our world come to?

"Fragrance free" is its own beast. Sometimes, it means that no artificial fragrance was added (which is good), but sometimes it means that chemicals were added to mask the product's natural odor (which is bad . . . very bad). They're trying to trick you into thinking it doesn't have a fragrance because none were added, but instead it really means that it has no fragrance because they added so much garbage to eliminate it. Sometimes they'll even use preservatives to mask odor, which means that the brand lists the preservative as a "fragrance" in the ingredient list to make it look like the product is preservative-free—how tricky! "Fragrance" can also show up in various forms like "parfum," "perfume," "aroma," and "flavor." The problem lies in the fact that the government doesn't legally require ingredients within the term "fragrance" to be listed so you have no idea what these fragrances are. They could be natural, but most likely they're artificial or synthetic. Another thing to keep in mind is if you see "fragrance" listed in the ingredients, it can actually contain hundreds of unlisted ingredients, which may or may not be harmful.

"Contains 99.9% . . ." These types of percentage statements imply that the product contains that exact percentage of the ingredient (for example: aloe vera). In reality, it's saying that the active ingredient is present. So, one drop of 99.9 percent aloe vera solution added to a face cleanser can still be listed as 99.9 percent aloe vera. Another tricky thing brands will do is put a lower percentage of an active ingredient. For instance, if it's been proven that 5 percent of tea tree oil was effective in a study, they may only add 1 percent.

Many companies also capitalize on words like "natural" or "organic" to imply that the entire product is natural or organic, when in reality, it's only present in very small amounts. I thought that this one deserved its own section, though, so we're going to talk about that next. Follow me.

Building a Natural Skincare Routine

"*Natural*" and "*organic*" products are very popular right now—and that's a good thing! I can only hope that this isn't a trend, but instead, a lifestyle that's here to stay. So, it's only "natural" (pun intended) that the skincare and makeup industry would follow suit. What you put in and on your body is super important; it can inextricably alter your health, the environment, and other living things. Plus, the things closest to its purest form in nature are likely to be the most beneficial—the universe equipped us with everything we need, don't you think?

Unfortunately, the FDA has pretty loose regulations when it comes to this as well, especially in the beauty industry. It's important to know the definitions of each so that you can accurately build a healthy skincare routine.

"Natural" can pretty much be plastered on any packaging. A natural ingredient is simply derived from nature as opposed to being made synthetically; that means it can be plant-, animal-, or mineral-based. The term can also be used for an ingredient regardless of how it was treated (which often involves unnatural chemicals as you can imagine). In fact, most ingredients have some degree of physical processing (heating, additives, etc.) or altering. Most "natural" products didn't jump straight from the farm into its biodegradable container. That's why health nuts often look for "raw" products—it means the ingredients haven't been treated with any kind of heat. Heat might not inherently sound bad—we all love hot showers, hot tubs, and steamy romances—but it can actually counteract the efficacy of many ingredients. When exposed to heat, many ingredients lose their important nutrients. What's the point in buying aloe vera aloe vera if it's not going to accurately do its job, right?

If you want your skincare to be natural and raw, you probably want it to be organic, too. The term "organic" specifically applies to plant ingredients that have been confirmed by a reputable agency like the USDA. Therefore, certified-organic ingredients must meet specific requirements to earn that seal of approval. More importantly, an ingredient can only be considered organic if the origin, production, and farming follow specific rules that facilitate safe environmental practices. So, if you see a product with a USDA Organic seal (or another certifying seal), you know that it contains over 95 percent organic ingredients and closely follows these rules. Unfortunately, the FDA does not specifically regulate the term "organic" when it comes to beauty or skincare products. But, if you're using things like body oils in your skincare routine (as you should be doing), this may help you. Not only should you be looking for organic products because they're better for your skin, but if a company takes the time to care about it in the first place, they're likely concerned with quality in all aspects of its production.

We've mentioned "synthetic" ingredients a few times without really defining what it means. Synthetic ingredients are ones not found in nature, but instead, usually made in a lab. However, they aren't always bad like they're made out to be. Truthfully, they can sometimes be safer than their natural counterparts. For example, L-ascorbic acid is a synthetic ingredient and it's actually more effective than it is in its natural form, which is vitamin C. So generally speaking, natural ingredients are better for you, but once again, you might need to do your research from time to time if you're unsure.

We know how to spot a vegan and cruelty-free label, but we don't know why they're important. It probably comes as no surprise that most of those who care about nature also care about animals. The reason why most products are tested on animals in the first place is because they contain ingredients that can be harmful to humans. So, their philosophy is "let's test it out on an animal first." I won't deluge you with information about animal cruelty, but if you don't know exactly what it is or how it works, I highly suggest researching it. It might convince you to look for that little leaping bunny on all of your packaging. Vegan products are free of animal by-products. Most animal by-products are not ideal for the human body. Using animal by-products is also one of the biggest contributors to global warming. Granted some products are controversial—I know vegans who support the use of beeswax—but generally speaking, I would stay away from non-vegan skincare. Caring about animals is a big part of building a healthy beauty routine. Thankfully, the industry seems to be moving in that direction as well.

Department Store vs. Drugstore

If I can bring back my dude Billy Shakespeare for a second to pose the eternal beauty dilemma: "to drugstore or not to drugstore, that is the question." You've all thought about it before. Do I splurge on the Bobbi Brown lipstick at Bloomingdale's or just get a similar one from Revlon? I grew up in a family that firmly believed that off-brand anything was just as good as high-end. I had other plans, though. I always believed (and still do) that things are more expensive for a reason. Of course, that's not always the case. Sometimes you're simply paying for good branding. But sometimes you are actually paying for better quality.

When it comes to skincare and makeup, mass-market brands tend to incorporate more synthetic and less expensive ingredients. Higher-end brands also tend to have more pigment, advanced chemistry, and expensive technologies to improve the quality of their product. High-end makeup also has cleaner ingredients, fewer fillers, and more diversity (both skin shade and skin needs).

Another major difference between department store and drugstore products is the quantity of ingredients. We kind of talked about this earlier with the aloe vera scenario. Just because a drugstore face cleanser has aloe vera in it doesn't mean that it has the same amount or efficiency as a department store version. Higher-end products are more likely to have a higher quantity of the beneficial ingredients. So even though you may look at them and say, "see, they both have aloe vera," they don't actually do the same job. Sometimes it's worth the splurge for quality.

Building on that, most products have base ingredients. In general, department store products tend to also have better quality base ingredients, which allow the products to possibly feel smoother, last longer, be gentler, etc. The ingredients have usually undergone more research and testing than drugstore brands. They also tend to have a lower water count (yes, water's important, but who wants to pay $59 for a vial of water?).

At the end of the day, you should only pay for what you can afford. If you can, choose quality of the product over quantity. Isn't it better to have one face cleanser that works beautifully than to try three or four that are all just okay? I think it's great to choose drugstore when you're experimenting with lip color, eye shadow, or even nail polish. But when it comes to your skin, you want to make sure you're using the best ingredients. Drugstore products are also less likely to be natural, organic, cruelty-free, vegan—and all those other important things we just talked about.

Don't buy skincare just because it's expensive, though. Do your research, find out what ingredients they're using, and make an executive decision on whether it's worth the splurge. No one said building a healthy skincare routine was easy! If you stick to better ingredients (no, this isn't a Papa John's ad), you will surely notice healthy, radiant skin. "Shall I compare thee to a summer's day?"

CHAPTER 7

Skincare— Who Needs It?

Skin is the largest organ of the body. It's also the first line of defense against bacteria and other bad stuff. Not to mention that clear (or not so clear) skin is usually one of the first things people notice about you. So, it only makes sense that you should want to take very good care of it. Most people, myself included, probably didn't start a proper skincare routine until it was already too late—that is, when you started getting pimples, sunburn, fine lines, etc. Not to say that starting a skincare regime say, in your teens is *too late* per se, but imagine if you had started even earlier.

Different ages require different products. If you're in your forties and are still using the exact same skincare routine as you did in your teens, it's time to switch things up. That's because a pimply teenager needs different ingredients than the aging skin of a sixty-year-old. Not to say that there's anything *wrong* with aging skin. In fact, skin ages like a fine wine. You cannot help the changes your skin goes through (well, perhaps you can stall them a bit) because there's no magic potion or wish-granting genie out there to prevent it from happening. So instead of being on a quest to constantly eradicate all signs of aging, the best thing you can do is take the absolute best care of what you've got. As cheesy as it sounds, beauty really does come from within . . . but, a little confidence with healthy skin never hurt anybody.

In Your Twenties

If each skincare decade had its own *Real Housewives* tagline, your twenties would be: "I love having fun, but I always make sure to use protection."

What? Not *that* kind of protection—although that is important, too. According to virtually every skincare expert, your twenties are all about forming good habits now to prevent damage in the future. The skin is at its peak in your twenties with fruitful collagen production and elastin. If you want that youthful glow later, you have to work hard to keep it.

When it comes to a skincare routine, keep it simple: cleanser, moisturizer, SPF. You'll likely want to have a morning and evening routine, too. If you're feeling proactive, you can also throw an exfoliant and antioxidant serum in the mix. Plus, I know I don't have to say this, but don't sleep in your makeup. Also, stay away from alcohol and make good dietary choices.

I know we've already discussed this ad nauseam, but the most important step of prevention is—drumroll please—sunscreen! This needs to be a part of your daily routine; it's the best way to prevent skin cancer and ensure radiant skin for years to come. After all, UV rays are responsible for 80 percent of visible signs of aging. If you don't want to douse yourself in beachy Hawaiian Tropic in the winter, find a lightweight sunscreen or moisturizer with built-in SPF. Just make sure it's always broad spectrum.

Your twenties are also probably a decade of acne breakouts. I know, you thought they'd be gone by now, but the reality is that many adults still get them. Due to hormonal shifts, the type of acne you get in your twenties tends to be on your cheeks and jawline. The treatments you were using in your teens might be too aggressive for this kind of acne, which means you'll need to switch to a less drying routine. The best thing you can do is wash your face with a gentle cleanser twice a day to restore your skin's natural oil production and minimize breakouts.

Follow that up with an oil-free moisturizer and a spot treatment infused with salicylic acid or benzoyl peroxide. A retinoid can also help with acne, hyperpigmentation, and wrinkles. Side note: collagen starts to break down in your mid-twenties and decreases about 1 percent each year after that. Yikes. So, you might not have any wrinkles yet, but you'll definitely want to start combating them now.

After cleanser comes the moisturizer. If your skin wasn't dry in your teens, it might be starting to dry out a bit now. We know moisturizer is important because it also helps your skin stay hydrated so that it can properly repair itself.

In Your Thirties

If your skincare routine in your thirties had a *Real Housewives* tagline, it would be: "I'm finally learning how to rid myself of past mistakes—with exfoliation, of course."

Your thirties are usually when the aging process begins: collagen starts to decline, leaving your skin thinner while sweat and oil glands slow down and dry it out.

As far as the basics go, not much changes. If you've been diligent with the sunscreen, you probably don't have too much damage. If you haven't already, try incorporating one with antioxidants. In terms of cleansers, you might want to try one with hydroxy acids to increase cell renewal. With moisturizers, now's the time to make sure you're using one with antioxidants and peptides. You could also try using a facial oil—not only does it add a youthful glow, but it plumps the skin to help temporarily reduce wrinkles.

Good news: your acne has likely subsided. Yay! Unfortunately, your complexion may start to dull because of slow cell turnover. The remedy? Exfoliation. Most dermatologists recommend exfoliating three to five times a week in your thirties to help remove dead skin cells and fight early signs of aging. Exfoliating can mean physical scrubs, chemical peels (AHAs are great), or a cleansing brush.

The bad news about your acne subsiding is that it's because your skin has started to dry out. Woohoo! You'll also start to notice some hyperpigmentation, fine lines, sun spots, dark circles, sagging eyelids, expression lines, and all that other fun stuff. Your skin might even feel less smooth and your pores will become enlarged. Melasma (pigment) may also form during pregnancy or as the result of genetic predisposition. Who said aging wasn't fun, am I right?

If you weren't using retinol in your twenties, you'll likely want to start now—and perhaps even get a prescription retinoid from your dermatologist. Retinol will help your skin build collagen, prevent wrinkles, and correct hyperpigmentation. More than thirty years of research proves this, too. Just make sure to follow up with a moisturizer to ensure it doesn't dry out your skin too much.

There's more on the market than just retinol, though. Niacinamide will help with undereye redness, hyaluronic acid will help with fine lines, and caffeine will prevent inflammation. Plus, let's not forget about antioxidants like vitamin C, vitamin E, and goji berry. Antioxidants are like fire extinguishers, coming in and putting out fires caused by the false invincibility of youth: hyperpigmentation, extinguished.

If the serums, creams, and exfoliants just aren't cutting it, now might be a time to look into treatments. Botox, used sparingly, can help prevent the deepening of wrinkles, while Fraxel can help reduce sunspots. You might also want to consider microdermabrasion, laser toning, and medium-depth chemical peels.

In Your Forties

Your forties skincare routine is the Sonja Morgan of *Housewives* taglines —fun and flirty: "When things get dry, I like to make a big splash . . . with moisture, that is." Basically, this decade is all about combating the hormonal effects of perimenopause (the phase right before menopause): collagen loss, fine lines, etc. The best way to do that is with extra moisture.

At this point, we know we need to wear sunscreen, but what you probably didn't know is that older cells are even more vulnerable to UV damage. Since your cell turnover has slowed down, it means sunscreen is a must. In terms of cleansers, keep it gentle, but you can now use one that's a bit more hydrating. While you're at it, you may as well use a super hydrating moisturizer, too. Look for ingredients like glycerin and ceramides. You should also try incorporating oils like yangu, marula, and passionfruit to lock in moisture. In your forties, there's a reduction of sebaceous oil, which means your skin loses its ability to hold onto moisture. Continue to exfoliate so that your serums and moisturizers can do their jobs.

Your forties are the decade to invest in products with active ingredients. The decrease in collagen and elastin means that there may be volume loss in your face. Hyperpigmentation will continue to get worse as well. This may seem like a train straight to hell that you can't stop, but it's really not that scary. Simply build on your existing routines with products that target specific concerns. You may have already started using retinol (or vitamin A) in your thirties (or twenties if you're proactive), but consider upping the dosage in your forties. It's a good investment in your nightly routine because it'll improve cell turnover and collagen production, as well as reduce acne for those still suffering from breakouts. Antioxidants are also a beautiful thing. Serums that are rich in vitamins will also help protect and repair your skin from sun damage—bonus points if you layer it under your night cream. Peptides, meanwhile, send messages to your cells to counteract aging and stimulate collagen. If you want to reduce those expression lines, peptides will do that. If you haven't started using an eye cream, this is your time; look for ones with those antioxidants or retinol we keep talking about. Makeup may also need to be altered during this time due to changes in skin texture and tone. Fear not! If you've been wanting to experiment with new products, aging is a good excuse—not like you really needed one, anyway.

Treatments in your forties aren't all that different from treatments in your thirties. Lasers may start to become your new BFF, though. Lasers can help tighten skin, fix broken capillaries, and banish hyperpigmentation. Botox can also start to make a big difference. Your forties are also a time to try deep chemical peels, if you're game.

In Your Fifties

Your fifties skincare routine *Real Housewives'* tagline would be: "I don't mind waiting in lines, but I do mind the ones on my face."

Or maybe you *don't* mind the ones on your face—and you shouldn't! However, it is a common concern for many women. In your fifties, those hormones we talked about in your forties have now drastically dropped due to menopause. This leads to a further breakdown of fat, muscle, and bone, which equates to volume loss (hello jowls), sagging (hello "turkey" neck), and wrinkles. It also leads to dryness so hydration is *key* in your fifties.

In terms of routine, skincare in your fifties is very similar to skincare in your forties. Keep your cleanser the same. With moisturizer, now's the time to look to ceramides for help. Skin becomes thinner in your fifties, which means that a lot of the fat that used to keep your skin looking smooth and supple is no longer there. Ceramides will lock in the moisture and give the appearance of plump and youthful skin. If you're not already using hyaluronic acid, that will help, too. In terms of retinol, some dermatologists recommend increasing your dosage while others think it can be too harsh in your fifties. You know your body best: if your skin is super dry, it's probably time to cut down on the retinol and just focus on moisturizing. Also, keep it up with the antioxidants, peptides, and eye cream.

In Your Sixties+

Your sixties and older *Real Housewives'* tagline is simple: "I never start fights, but I've become an expert at fighting signs of aging."

In your sixties, signs of aging are going to happen at a more pronounced rate. You'll start noticing vertical wrinkles around your mouth and loss of volume in the lips. This is also the time when precancerous moles or skin cancer are more likely to manifest. Once you reach your seventies, your skin will look more translucent and feel kind of dry and crepe-y. I think it's safe to say most of us prefer our crepes with Nutella and whipped cream.

Not much has changed from the previous two decades in terms of routine: (super) gentle cleanser, antioxidant serum, facial oil, moisturizer, SPF, retinol . . . you know the drill. At this point, you'll definitely want to incorporate botanical extracts or intense moisturizers if you haven't already. Look for ingredients like shea nut butter and hyaluronic acid to do the trick.

In Your Teens

Okay, let's backtrack a bit. I know after discussing crepe-y skin, your teens probably sound like a breeze. But let's take a moment to reflect, shall we? If your tween/teen years were anything like mine, they were most likely filled with Ne-Yo songs, unrequited crushes, and acne . . . lots and lots of acne. Clean & Clear and Neutrogena didn't quite cut it for me—although those commercials with Vanessa Hudgens cheerfully splashing water in her face were highly convincing. In fact, I remember *praying* for the days of wrinkles just so I wouldn't have to keep experimenting with the latest topical prescriptions and popping Accutane pills like Tic Tacs. How could I have so much acne at fifteen years old but not have experienced a single pimple only a few years before?

Your oil glands shut off when you're about six months old and are only activated again when stimulated by the hormones of puberty—(cue the ominous music). In fact, acne is usually the first sign of puberty. Before that, life is simple. You can wash your face . . . or not . . . whatever . . . it doesn't matter. You'll still wake up looking like an angel the next day. Once you start getting breakouts, though, it can be hard to keep them at bay. We often dive into spot treatments, but those can often be too harsh and drying. Instead, retinoids like Differin (or other all-over topical treatments) are a much better alternative. If you're experiencing severe cystic acne, there's most likely a much larger issue at hand. Once I cut out all animal products from my diet and switched to an all-natural skincare routine, my skin cleared up like you wouldn't believe. But when in doubt, a dermatologist will know the right products and treatments to alleviate it.

Before rushing to the intense acne products (or assuming that you even have acne at all), comes cleansing. As a teen it's super important to wash your face before bed. Your sebum production is high which can clog up your pores—plus, think about how many times you get nervous throughout the day as a teen: walking past your crush, getting called on by your teacher to answer an impossible algebra question, having to run the mile in gym class. Cleansing in the morning is less important but should probably be done if you have the time. A classic mistake most teens make (me) is using a soap instead of a cleanser. Remember, soaps tend to have higher pH levels, unlike the natural pH of your skin. Cleansers are more neutral and therefore less irritating. Another helpful trick is keeping cleansing wipes in your backpack—especially if they have salicylic acid in them. They're perfect post workout, awkward run-in, etc.

You didn't think I would forget about the sunscreen, did you? It's never too early to start. If you've just started wearing makeup, find a tinted moisturizer or foundation with SPF to supplement the sunscreen I hope you're already wearing on a daily basis.

Skincare for Kids
Not to be confused with Kars4Kids.

This might seem like a silly category considering most kids probably don't have a skincare routine. Although I do like the visual of a three-year-old lumbering out of bed, dragging herself to the bathroom, globbing on way too much moisturizer (the kind with a Disney princess on the front of the bottle), and haphazardly applying blush and some lipstick before running out the door because she has an expense report due at noon. Whether you have kids or are one yourself (kudos to you for selecting this book instead of *Twilight*), there are some things you should know about taking care of youthful skin.

For starters, one misconception about children's skincare is that they need to be bathed every day. In fact, The American Academy of Dermatology says children ages six to twelve only need to be bathed once or twice a week. Even babies don't need to be bathed every day— although your baby's food and vomit spills may say otherwise. Too much bathing can dry out the skin and lead to eczema. Plus, they need that good bacteria. So, go ahead, live like the French do—and pick up a baguette while you're at it.

While we're on the topic of bad things for children's skin, you should definitely stay away from those horrifying, unpronounceable chemical ingredients (not the Latin kind). Children's skin is about 30 percent thinner than adults and it absorbs most of what it comes in contact with. Plus, the blood-brain battier that blocks chemicals from seeping into the brain tissues is not fully formed until a baby is six months old. Basically, carcinogens are ten times more potent for babies (and some are even sixty-five times more potent) than for adults. Again, it would be super cool if the FDA could regulate that stuff better, but until they do, I have to inform you myself. In fact, it has been found that 77 percent of ingredients in 17,000 reviewed children's products have never been assessed for safety. On average, children are exposed to twenty-seven skincare products that have not been found safe for them. Diaper wipes alone often contain chemicals found in antifreeze, preservatives, and perfume. This can seriously cause long-term damage and harm their reproductive system!

If you're wondering what skincare routine is ideal for children, here's a guideline broken down by age . . .

- **Two to Five Years Old**: Now's a good time to teach them the importance of washing their hands (and face). Not only because I (someone who's not a relative) don't want to touch their boogers, but because it will help them stay healthy. Use a gentle wash for their baths followed by a lightweight lotion.
- **Six to Nine Years Old**: This is a good time to introduce them to a proper skincare routine. Nothing too crazy, of course. Just a gentle facial cleanser, toner, and lightweight lotion.
- **Ten to Twenty Years Old**: This is when you introduce the separate morning and nighttime routines—perhaps even an exfoliant a couple nights a week. Stay on track with the gentle cleanser, toner, and lotion.

CHAPTER 8

The Bare Necessities

We're all fascinated by the inside of people's medicine cabinets. When you pull back that mirrored door above the bathroom sink, you never know what you may find: a rusty nail clipper, mysterious medication, vitamin C cream from that trendy new brand that you and your friend hated on together, so why the heck does she have it in her medicine cabinet?! Basically, they can tell us a lot about a person and their unique habits. Some people even make a point of snooping through them in strange homes—while others simply open up theirs willingly to *Into the Gloss*. Pro tip: snooping can also lead to some unwanted discoveries, like your parents "massage dice," so snoop with caution.

I know what you're thinking. I, too, was hoping this "Bare Necessities" chapter would be about *The Jungle Book*, but alas, this is a skincare book, so instead it's about the must-have items in your medicine cabinet—plus, Mowgli spent his entire life outside and never once even applied SPF, so you probably shouldn't be getting your skincare advice from him anyway. While it's true that not everyone has the same exact items inside their medicine cabinet, there are some general products that are good to have. Think of this as your grocery list of skincare items. Whether you're a beginner, full-blown skincare addict, or somewhere in between, there's a meal (skincare) plan for everyone.

The Essentials

Let's just say you're only allowed to have three skincare items—or maybe you only *want* three skincare items (#minimalism). What do you think they should be? As with everything in life, it depends who you ask. You could also argue that you have different needs for morning and evening so the three products you need might differ depending on the time of day.

I think most experts would agree that cleanser, moisturizer, and sunscreen are the three essentials.

- **Cleansers**: Cleansers get all of the dirt, debris, and oil off your face so that you have a clean canvas. Cleansing will also help prepare your face to receive the benefits of the products you'll use afterward. You may as well throw out the other products if you're not going to cleanse beforehand—unless they're expensive, then just donate to a friend in need (me). Since the skin on your face is more delicate than the rest of your body, a bar of soap simply isn't good enough. A cleanser should also be strong enough to remove the bad bacteria, while being gentle enough to keep the good bacteria. You really should be cleansing twice a day. In the morning you might be thinking, *but my face only touched my pillow, what gives*? But you'll want to remove any residual night cream, makeup, or impurities from the previous day. You don't want dull skin and breakouts, do you? You can even double cleanse to be extra thorough. A dime-sized amount of cleanser, fifteen seconds of massaging, and warm water usually does the trick.
- **Moisturizers**: Moisturizers hydrate and soften the skin by preventing water loss from the outer layers of the skin. It also acts as a barrier against irritants. This is probably the one product that all dermatologists would recommend using year-round for all skin types. The best part is that you can find moisturizers

for every skin type, season, and budget. Not only does skin lose moisture after cleansing, but as we age, it loses the ability to retain moisture as well. Of course, you'll want one with broad-spectrum sunscreen protection during the day. Some even have antiaging and restorative properties, meaning you can forgo the serums if you'd like. For nighttime, use a thicker, richer formula—possibly even one with collagen and elastin. You just need a dime-sized amount for the face and neck before lightly massaging it into the skin.

- **Sunscreens**: Sunscreens are the best way to prevent aging skin, brown spots, wrinkles, and cancer—a jack-of-all-trades, really. All experts unanimously agree that it's the most important product you can use on your skin every day. In fact, melanoma (skin cancer) is the biggest cause of cancer death among people in their twenties. This is why you need it in your medicine cabinet! If you use a chemical sunscreen, apply it after cleansing (before applying your other products). If you use a physical sunscreen, apply it after your moisturizer and other products. They even make sheer and invisible gel sunscreens so it will dry clear and won't even feel like you're wearing one. If you're lazy in the morning, find a moisturizer with an SPF of at least 30—killing two birds with one stone.

The Intermediate

I would imagine most people reading this book fall within this category. It seems to be the Goldilocks sweet spot of "not too few," "not too many," but "just right." After all, you want to treat yourself and your skin, without spending too much time or money on a routine. Naturally, you should still keep the cleanser, moisturizer, and SPF in there, but you'll also want to incorporate some extras.

- **Cleanser**
- **Toner**: Toner helps balance, clean, calm, and exfoliate the skin. Tap water and other formulations can throw your skin's natural pH out of whack, so a toner is *great* for that. You'll notice that your skin appears clearer and softer. Toner is also wonderful for removing excess dirt, makeup, oil, and pollution. I know what you're thinking: *isn't my cleanser supposed to do that*? Yes, but cleanser (even double cleansing) is not perfect. Toner can also help exfoliate and calm the skin—especially if you're prone to skin conditions like eczema. It may even help minimize pores. Sure, a lot of experts consider toner to be optional. Some people also have a negative connotation with the word because it reminds them of the harsh formulations from the '80s. Toners have evolved to be much less harsh. Some ingredients to look for include: AHAs, BHAs, hyaluronic acid, rose water, green tea, and vitamins. Apply a toner after cleansing and before putting on any other products. Use a cotton pad and simply wipe it over the face. Side note: you don't need a super expensive toner to get the job done. I use diluted apple cider vinegar that I bought at my grocery store for like $6 and it works beautifully.
- **Exfoliants**: Exfoliants slough off dead skin cells and help speed up the production of new ones. They also help unclog pores to prevent acne and allow for deeper penetration of other products. This may sound like it should be the job of a cleanser, which is why some people choose not to exfoliate, but it is definitely that extra step missing in your routine. As we know, the skin renewal process slows down as we age, so exfoliating a few times a week can help create radiant skin. If mechanical exfoliants (scrubs) are too intense, try a chemical one instead.
- **Serums**: Serums have more active ingredients that are designed to address specific concerns like pigmentation, acne, wrinkles, etc. Some people think a moisturizer is enough to do the trick,

which is why they prefer not to use a serum. Unlike a moisturizer, though, a serum is highly concentrated and penetrates deeper into the skin to deliver nutrients. If you don't have too many skin concerns, you can also use a serum to protect from free radicals that come from sun damage and pollution. Look for ingredients like hyaluronic acid, retinol, antioxidants, peptides, or niacinamide depending on your skincare needs—you can even use multiple formulas. Just don't try mixing it with your moisturizer to save time—you'll actually lessen its ability to absorb effectively. Simply apply it one by one, serum first. Also, a little goes a long way! No need to apply a dollop like it's sour cream on Taco Tuesday.

- **Moisturizer**
- **Eye Cream**: Eye cream is a moisturizer formulated for the sensitive area around your eyes. Your eye area is more prone to wrinkles and has fewer oil glands, so sometimes it needs some extra TLC. Sure, you might not *need* eye cream, but it can help with a youthful appearance. Raccoons are cute AF but I certainly don't want to look like one, you know? Best of all, there are different eye creams for different concerns: antioxidants for wrinkles, caffeine for puffy eyes, vitamin K and kojic acid for dark circles. Gently pat it (most people use their ring finger because it's the gentlest) along your ocular bone. Experts usually recommend applying it before your moisturizer, but I don't know that it matters all that much.
- **Sunscreen**

The Expert

- **Cleanser**
- **Cleansing Tools**: Cleansing tools make your cleanser work even better. The first thing that probably comes to mind is a Clarisonic device, but some people prefer washcloths, LED light

therapy, or toning devices. You basically just want something that will help remove impurities for a smoother, clearer complexion. Some people find these tools too abrasive, so you may not want to incorporate it into your everyday routine. It's good to keep in your medicine cabinet for those days when you want a little extra help.

- **Toner**
- **Exfoliants**
- **Acne Treatment**: Acne treatment helps with acne. If you don't need this step then you are so lucky and congratulations on your good genes. Perhaps you get the occasional pimple, though—we all do, right? I think this is something everyone should keep in their medicine cabinet . . . just in case. A topical treatment with benzoyl peroxide is usually a safe bet. Simply dab it on any pimples (or spots you foresee turning into a pimple) and watch it disappear (or at least reduce in size). P.S. most modern toothpastes don't work for pimples anymore, so you might actually have to splurge on a legitimate treatment for this one. If harsh chemicals scare you though, you can go the natural route with essential oils like tea tree—this can sometimes be too harsh for the skin, but in moderation it works wonders (like dabbing it on a pimple, for example).
- **Serum**
- **Masks**: Masks can serve many functions. Masks can assist with cleansing in that they can remove dirt and oil from the pores. Many of them are also similar to serums in that they are highly concentrated and target specific concerns like acne, wrinkles, hyperpigmentation, dullness, etc. Also, unlike toners and serums, masks deliver ingredients under occlusion, which helps the ingredients absorb better. You might not want to use a mask every day, but it's something useful to keep in your medicine cabinet for those times when you have a last-minute event and are looking for

an extra boost. In the past few years, the popularity of masks has skyrocketed—Sephora alone has more than 400 varieties.

- **Moisturizer**
- **Eye Cream**
- **Face Oils**: Face oils have many benefits including hydrating, brightening, disinfecting, and calming the skin. When choosing face oils, it's best to stick to essential or carrier oils or those without added fragrance because we know that the purest route

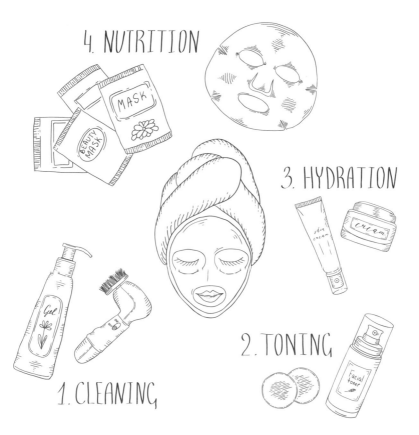

is the best route. Some of these you may already have in your medicine (or kitchen) cabinet: olive oil, rose hip oil, lavender. One of the best things about facial oils is that they're made without water—most skincare products have water listed as the first ingredient—so, you know you're getting a high concentration of really good stuff for your skin; stuff that will likely help with that "natural" glow we're all trying to achieve. Twice a day, apply it after your serum but before your moisturizer—it'll help lock in the benefits of the serum and prep your skin for the cream. A dime-sized amount should be just enough to get that ethereal glow without looking like a glazed doughnut or marathon runner.

- **Sunscreen**

CHAPTER 9

Classics and Trends

Similar to falling in love, eating cheese, or watching those pimple-popping videos on YouTube, the discovery of a new skincare ingredient or product is a highly addictive experience. It holds so much hope and promise. Surely retinol will cure my acne! Not completely. Okay, what about hyaluronic acid? No, that didn't totally work, either.

Trends can be fun and super effective. Sometimes, though, it's best to rely on the classics. Think about the stuff your grandma used. Sure, not all of it was great—lead-infused products weren't our finest moment as a society—but many products are in fact classics for a reason . . . because they work. Other times, it's best to fall back on the basics, like ingredients you can find in your kitchen—they come from nature so your skin is bound to love it.

If you just can't get enough of those new products, though, there are some you should probably know about (or perhaps you already do). Fortunately for you, the skincare world is constantly evolving and there are always new trends on the horizon.

The Classics

It's hard to go wrong with classics. Just think about how many brands have built a reputation around it: Ray-Bans, Corvette, Coca-Cola. Classics are reliable, simple, and trusted, which is why they're still used today. In case you didn't have a savvy mom or grandma to teach you, here are some of the more popular ones you should know about:

- **Pond's Cold Cream**: All right, let's start with the holy grail of classic skincare items. I still use Pond's to this day. My mom introduced me to it when I first started wearing makeup because she uses it. She started using it because my grandma 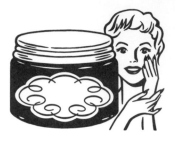 used it. See how that works? Side note: does anyone else remember that episode of *Mad Men* where they have to come up with an ad for Pond's? That's how much of an iconic product it is (actually, it's been around for over 150 years). Most people love Pond's because it's inexpensive and really cuts through makeup—I've found that makeup wipes, micellar waters, and oils just don't work as well. With Pond's you can glob it on, gently wipe with a tissue, and have very little residue left on your face. Plus, it doesn't clog your pores and is great for sensitive skin. It can also be used as a moisturizer—it's super hydrating without being too heavy or sticky. Some people even use it as a mask, makeup primer, or body lotion.
- **Aquaphor**: Aquaphor is basically a cure-all petroleum jelly product. Chapped lips? Aquaphor. Dry hands? Aquaphor. Impromptu makeup illuminator? Aquaphor. My college roommate recommended it to me (her dad was a dermatologist) and I've never looked back. I can't even imagine using another product on my lips. Aquaphor is super hydrating and has never caused me any irritation. Plus, it's apparently safe enough for babies.
- **Clinique Dramatically Different Moisturizing Lotion**: I don't have any experience with this product, but it's a cult classic with one bottle sold every fifteen seconds. Evelyn Lauder, dermatologist Norman Orentreich, and *Vogue* editor Carol

Phillips launched Clinique in 1968 with the mission to convince others that good skin was not just a matter of genetics, but could in fact be created. They launched their famous 3-Step Skincare System, which included the Dramatically Different Moisturizing Lotion. It has a recognizable yellow bottle that you may have seen in your mom's medicine cabinets. Fifty years later, the formula has remained the same, with the first three ingredients after water being mineral oil, glycerin, and petrolatum. It's not always a favorite of dermatologists because it lacks a lot of the modern-day ingredients that optimize hydration levels (hello, hyaluronic acid), but it's still a classic nonetheless.

- **Dove Beauty Bar**: Dove's Beauty Bar is one of the most recognizable soap bars (cue the Kanye voice) of all time. It was created in 1957 and has become a classic for its ability to clean without making your skin too dry. In fact, sixty of them are sold every second—tickets to a Beyoncé concert are the only thing I can think of that might sell just as quickly. I was a loyal follower for many years (of Dove that is) before deciding to take a more natural approach.

- **Vaseline**: Vaseline is similar to Aquaphor in that it's a cure-all petroleum jelly product. Created in 1892, it's remained a skincare classic for many reasons: it heals wounds, hydrates skin, repairs chapped lips, reduces eczema, softens callouses—the list goes on and on. It's probably the one skincare product I used regularly as a kid; I imagine I'm not the only one. Although petroleum jelly is controversial, it is a great occlusive, which is why it's also sometimes also used for patch-testing and locking in perfume fragrance. Studies have even shown that Vaseline promotes cellular healing without the risk of allergic reaction, making it better than Neosporin. Although I definitely would not recommend slathering it on your face (unless you love acne breakouts), Marilyn Monroe claimed to do just that in order to maintain her clear complexion. She used it as a moisturizer, highlighter, and even primer. If it's good enough for Marilyn . . .

- **Olay Moisturizing Lotion/Oil of Olay**: I bet this is another product you've seen in your mom's medicine cabinet. Created in 1949, Oil of Olay lotion was an immediate game changer because of its lightweight, fluid texture. The company eventually shortened the name to "Olay" and changed the lotion's formulation a bit.

- **Johnson's Baby Oil**: Created in 1938, Johnson's Baby Oil has proved itself as a useful skincare product that's not just for post-baby baths. Use it as a makeup remover, cuticle oil, or even shaving cream. Your skin will feel as soft and smooth as a baby's. Plus, it smells so clean and refreshing.

- **Nivea Crème**: Hitting the market in 1911, Nivea Crème considers itself the "mother of all modern creams." Its formula has pretty much remained the same but does include irritating preservatives with super long and scary names (not the all-natural Latin kind). Most dermatologists actually recommend staying away from it—especially those with eczema or a sensitivity to fragrance. Nonetheless, it's apparently Kate Middleton's go-to product and she looks pretty radiant.

- **Cetaphil Daily Facial Cleanser**: For many people, Cetaphil Daily Facial Cleanser was their first foray into the world of skincare. Ideal for acne and dry skin, it's gentle, effective, and doesn't strip your skin of its natural oils. It doesn't hurt that it's also pretty inexpensive and can be found at pretty much any and all drugstores. Your friends and dermatologists have probably both recommended it to you at some point.

- **Witch Hazel**: Witch hazel has been around since the nineteenth century, but its popularity resurged in the skincare world over the past few years. A natural antioxidant, it's renowned for its restorative properties and reducing inflammation, cellular damage, swelling, acne, eczema, sunburn, and wounds. Most people use it as a toner to help clean pores and get rid of excess oil without drying the skin. Some brands like Thayer's have even created formulas that are infused with ingredients like lavender and cucumber for added freshness.

Made in the Kitchen

Surely some of your best skincare experiences started in the kitchen. You probably prepared a gooey concoction of bananas, honey, and egg yolk with your best friends at a sleepover in middle school. Perhaps you still even run to the pantry when you're having a breakout or some excruciating sunburn. Natural is often the best way to go and was usually the first line of action before all of these fancy skincare ingredients were created. Here are some ingredients you can use:

- **Extra-Virgin Olive Oil**: the secret ingredient many Mediterranean women have been using for centuries to get shiny hair and radiant skin. Many people use it as a makeup remover. It's antibacterial and emollient, so you can literally apply it anywhere . . . and sop up the remainders with a fresh loaf of bread to funnel into your mouth.
- **Honey**: helps wounds heal faster, reduces scars, and just generally helps smooth your skin. Pretty much any at home face mask recipe you'll find includes honey. Make sure it's organic and skip out on ones that have "Bunches of Oats" or "Cheerios" at the end.
- **Steel-cut Oatmeal**: a personal breakfast favorite (topped with pumpkin seeds, banana slices, and cinnamon, of course), but it's also so good for your skin—which is why a lot of products are formulated with colloidal oatmeal. Toss some into your bath to relieve itching or irritation. Your skin will feel so soft and smooth afterward.

- **Egg Whites**: help combat oily skin and fight wrinkles. Simply whisk one raw egg white and apply it to your face until it dries. You'll also see them in a lot of at-home face mask recipes.
- **Coconut Oil**: an intensely hydrating skin treatment that can also be used as a makeup remover. Name one woman who hasn't tried coconut oil in the last five years, I dare you. If you're looking for a more holistic approach, this is a great option. However, it usually needs to be melted before use and has been known to clog pores. Although it might not be for everyone, it's worth giving a shot.
- **Yogurt**: contains lactic acid, making it one of the best exfoliating skin softeners. It can also help alleviate the sting of sunburn, as some of us learned the hard way circa 2002 in the Dominican Republic. Never forget.
- **Bayer**: saves more than just lives—it also saves skin. Aspirin can help reduce redness and puffiness, making it a great anti-acne mask. Crush it up, mix it with water, slap it on a pimple, and watch it shrink.
- **Black Tea**: alleviates the pain of sunburn. Allow it to soak into a towel before placing it on the sunburn. Feel the sting dissipate.
- **Oil and Vinegar**: a simple recipe for controlling acne. Not to be confused with salt and vinegar. Those are for your Lay's.
- **Sea Salt/Sugar**: are great for exfoliating the skin and are much safer than commercial exfoliators which often contain harsh chemicals.
- **Vegetable Shortening**: makes a great hand moisturizer and helps soften calluses. Try rubbing some on your heels and putting on a pair of socks before going to bed.
- **Aloe**: a go-to for sunburn but it can also be used to relieve inflammation, acne, and wounds. The enzymes in the plant even act as a gentle exfoliant. Before use, it makes a chic decoration in your bathroom.

- **Milk**: soothes and hydrates the skin. It can also help slough off dead skin cells thanks to lactic acid. Combined with other ingredients (like honey), it can keep acne at bay.
- **Apple Cider Vinegar**: is a great toner and acne treatment. If you find the sting to be a bit abrasive, dilute it with water. I love this stuff for a brighter and softer complexion.
- **Avocado**: is not just for Instagramming with toast. The fats and antioxidants in them can help keep your skin hydrated and reduce redness and irritation. Scoop it off your skin with tortilla chips and voila, you have a night of #selfcare.
- **Watermelon**: is surprisingly hydrating. Although it's 93 percent water, the remainder consists of antioxidants that help tone the skin, build collagen, and delay signs of aging. Ancient Egyptians used to actually mix watermelon extract with rosewater and sugar to create a moisturizer.
- **Turmeric**: is an antioxidant with anti-inflammatory and antibacterial properties. Yes, it tastes delicious in your Indian cuisine, but it also does wonders for your skin like clearing acne, wounds, eczema, and redness. It's a super powerful herb and has very strong coloring, so it can unfortunately dye the skin.

Turmeric Face Mask
- 1 teaspoon turmeric (use a little less if you're pale)
- 1 teaspoon honey
- 1 teaspoon Greek/natural yogurt
- 1 teaspoon lemon juice (optional)

Mix turmeric and honey in a bowl and add the yogurt until the mixture reaches the desired consistency. Add the lemon juice if using. Apply evenly over the face and leave on for 15–20 minutes. Just be careful not to spill any on your clothing or furniture—the turmeric will stain things!

Avocado-Honey Moisturizer
- 3 tablespoons fresh cream
- ¼ avocado (flesh only)
- 1 tablespoon honey

Place all three ingredients in a blender and puree into a smooth cream. Apply it to your skin and leave on for at least an hour. Rinse off with warm water.

Almond-Sugar Facial Scrub
- 3 tablespoons fresh cream
- 1 cup white sugar
- ½ cup brown sugar
- ½ cup ground almonds
- 2 tablespoons olive oil

Mix all ingredients well. Apply to dry face in a circular motion. Wash your face off with warm water, followed by cold water. Pat your face dry. Place in a jar and store in your refrigerator for future use.

Oatmeal-Honey Gentle Skin Cleanser
- 2 tablespoons oats
- 1 tablespoon plain yogurt
- ½ tablespoon honey

Mix all the ingredients in a bowl. Massage mixture into the skin and leave it for 5 minutes before rinsing with warm water.

Lemon Acne Spot Treatment
- A pinch of brewer's yeast
- A squeeze of lemon juice
- A bit of water

Okay, these measurements aren't wonderful but it's a spot treatment so you really only need to make as much as you'll use. Mix all of the ingredients together to make a paste. Apply it on the blemish and leave it for 10 minutes before rinsing with warm water. The yeast will fight bacteria and the lemon will dry out the pimple.

Trends

Classics are trusty and reliable, but trends are fresh and exciting. A new ingredient that will improve my skin tone? Brand packaging in millennial pink? The promise of eternal youth? Sign me up. It's so easy to get sucked in, especially when everyone else is jumping on the bandwagon. Some trends are great and end up sticking around, while others are just, well, trends. Luckily, current trends are gravitating more toward natural ingredients. Brands and consumers are realizing the importance of what mother nature already offers. Here are some that you've probably seen a lot of over the past couple of years:

Charcoal: You might have the visual of a summer barbecue or artists' palette, but the charcoal we use on our skin is slightly different.

The charcoal we use on our skin is heated to a high temperature first to increase absorption—it's also known as "activated charcoal." When placed on the face, it absorbs the oil and dirt from your pores. When you wash it off, the oil and dirt come off with it. This makes it a great treatment for those who suffer from acne. Charcoal has actually been used since ancient times, but has made a recent resurgence in the skincare world, especially with cleansers and masks. Some people describe charcoal as working like a magnet (and it kind of does), but just beware that many skincare products are formulated with a small amount. So, it might work like less of a magnet and more of a low-powered hand vacuum.

Rose: "I'll never let go, Jack"—of the intense hydration, that is. Rose-infused products are everywhere lately: facial mists, serums, toners, creams. In fact, according to a 2018 study, out of the top one-hundred toners/astringents in the skincare category, sixteen of them were infused with roses, which was a sizeable increase from just two months prior. Roses aren't a new thing, though. In fact, rosewater has been a staple in the Middle East for centuries. Roses are simply making a comeback because of their beneficial properties. First off, rose hips are super rich in antioxidants like vitamin C, E, D, A, and B3, which make them anti-inflammatory, hydrating, and ideal for calming redness and breakouts. Rose hip oil has also become really popular because it makes your skin super glowy, while brightening skin tone and fighting signs of aging. So, if you thought rose-themed products were limited to quartz facial rollers and pretty product packaging, you'd be wrong. The skincare industry likes to milk a trend for everything it's worth.

Vitamin C: You've heard so much about vitamin C at this point that you could probably tell *me* about it. Sure, vitamin C is really good for your body—it boosts the immune system, fights infections, increases collagen production, and repairs tissues—but it's also great for your skin. Vitamin C helps brighten skin, fade acne scars, reduce the signs of aging, and protect the skin from free radicals. In 2018, Pinterest actually reported that the searches for vitamin C skincare products had skyrocketed 3,379 percent. I'm pretty sure even sliced bread wasn't that popular. Vitamin C is also safe for pretty much all skin types and all times of day—it can actually increase the efficacy of your other products. I don't see this trend going anywhere for a while.

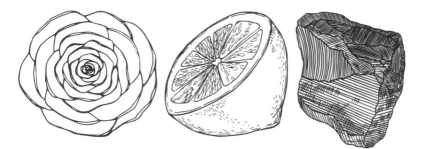

The Future of Skincare

This might sound ambiguous and clichéd, but the future of skincare has already begun. Some projected future trends have actually started trickling into the mainstream skincare industry, which is why I contemplated putting them in the above category. However, they haven't quite taken the industry by storm yet, and you are guaranteed to see a lot more of them in the next year or so:

Natural/Organic/Vegan/Cruelty-Free/Sustainable: You get the gist—healthy, ethical, plant-based products. Brand transparency has become super important to consumers. As a result, brands are giving more consideration to ingredients, packaging, and sourcing. With people embracing healthier and more active lifestyles, they want ingredients that nourish their body from the inside out and are free from harsh chemicals. Reports also show a large increase in sales with vegan and cruelty-free skincare products, especially among younger consumers. In fact, plant stem cells and marine biotechnology are believed to be the future of skincare. Plant stem cells specifically can be used to target wrinkles, visible capillaries, and sun damage. There is also expected to be a greater shift toward plant-based packaging (and away from plastic) and less water use in the supply chain. A lot of your favorite new brands might already be doing this, but it will likely become a consumer expectation in years to come.

Customization and Personalization: In modern times, the word "luxury" is synonymous with "individuality." No one wants to squeeze into one-size-fits-all clothing, so why would they want one-size-fits-all beauty? This is a particularly positive trend because it will hopefully become more inclusive of different skin tones and types. In fact, a recent study showed that 40 percent of makeup users in the United States felt frustrated by the lack of products out there that match their skin tone. Generally speaking, we also like to think of ourselves as unique and want brands that cater to that: "bespoke beauty," let's call it. Some brands are even using technology to find and create the perfect foundation based on your specific skin shade.

Cannabis: This is a fun one to write about. The stigma (and laws) surrounding cannabis have drastically decreased in recent years, which has led to an influx of research on its effects on the body. Although widely acknowledged for its medicinal properties, beauty brands have begun to capitalize on the benefits as well. CBD is known for its anti-inflammatory properties and ability to diminish acne and wrinkles. It can also help strengthen tissue, balance hormones, and rejuvenate skin cells. You've probably already noticed some of your favorite beauty brands incorporating this hero ingredient into everything from lip balm to eyebrow gel to foot cream. Expect to see much more of it in the future.

Anti–Blue Light: Blue light comes from digital devices like cell phones, tablets, and computers—so we are all exposed to it incessantly. Blue light is known to have similar effects to UV rays: wrinkles, pigmentation, etc. Brands are taking note of this concern and incorporating preventative measures into skincare—sunscreens specifically. The Asian market has been incorporating this technology into their skincare for a while, but the US market has just begun following suit. In the next few years, it will likely be everywhere.

Genderless Branding: Brands are becoming much more conscious of gender blurring barriers and are therefore beginning to promote unisex beauty. Some mainstream brands like CoverGirl and Maybelline have even signed male ambassadors, while a lot of newer brands use neutral packaging, labels, and marketing. Either way, this is another positive movement in the skincare industry. People of all genders, sizes, races, and religions have skin. Therefore, skincare shouldn't cater to one specific type of person. Skincare is meant to be inclusive, and the industry is finally getting the memo. Hopefully there are many good things to come in the future.

Acknowledgments

I would like to first and foremost thank Melissa Edwards for giving me this opportunity. This book was your brainchild and you simply allowed me to bring it to life. I still can't believe you trusted me (a naïve 23-year-old at the time) to take on such a big project. This came at a time in my life when I really needed it. I hope I've made you proud.

I would also like to thank Alison Fargis and everyone else at Stonesong for taking a chance on me.

Next, I have to thank my editor Leah Zarra at Skyhorse Publishing. Thank you for believing in this book and allowing my voice to shine through—in a much more polished way, of course. I appreciate your patience in manually combing through the manuscript to individually edit each and every em-dash that I wrote incorrectly.

I, of course, would be nowhere in life without my family. Ben, thank you for always supporting me, making me laugh, and keeping me humble; I deserve to be taken down a few notches every now and then. Mom, thank you for all of the sacrifices you've made for your children to be happy. You are without a doubt my biggest cheerleader, especially when it comes to my writing. I promise I will do everything in my power to become "the next David Sedaris." Dad, I give you lots of sass but truthfully, this opportunity would have never been possible if it weren't for you. Not only are you incredibly supportive, but you've connected me with lots of people over the years, which has led to lots of cool gigs—like this book! There isn't enough that I could say to aptly thank you both for everything that you've done for me over the past twenty-five years. I know your response would be, "reimburse us for your college tuition," but I doubt this book will gross even a fraction of that, so a simple, "I love you" will have to suffice.

You didn't think I would forget my dogs, did you? Thank you to all eight dogs we've had throughout my lifetime. You have each shaped me and how I've learned to love. You will forever be more important to me than any human that ever walks into my life.

I may not have even pursued writing in college had it not been for my high school English teacher Mary Ellen Phelan. Thank you for making us read the *New York Times* every Sunday and forcing us to write three-page papers daily on top of the other work you assigned. If it weren't for you, I never would have never known who Nicholas Kristof is and certainly would not have gone through my angsty Ayn-Rand-appreciation-phase. You tirelessly refined my craft and made me the writer I am today. Had you not guided me toward this path, I would be an interior designer still struggling to figure out CAD software.

Thank you to my NYU professors who in any way may have shaped my love and knowledge of fashion, beauty, and writing. If you want to include my book as mandatory syllabus reading, that would be greatly appreciated.

Thank you to my former coworkers and superiors (well, the ones I liked). You helped nurture my career, keep me sane, and even allowed me to try out comedy material at inappropriate times.

I have some supportive friends I want to acknowledge, even if I don't always talk to them on a regular basis: Jacqueline, Allison, Dylan, Anna, Kristin, Molly, and Francine. I've shouted you out in a book, so now you can't flake on our plans ever again.

I also have to acknowledge any relatives, friends of relatives, friends of friends, etc., who bought this book in support. Aunts, uncles, cousins, people my parents know—thank you.

Lastly, thank you to any ex-boyfriend or belligerent boss (you know who you are). You've fueled my rage-filled desire for success.

Hopefully this is just the beginning. I still have a lot of work to do before my *Barrel Fever* big break. Stay tuned.

Index

fifties, 92
foot care, 57–58
formaldehyde, 76–77
forties, 90–92
fragrance-free, 81
fragrances, 72, 77–78
Fraxel, 22–23, 90

G

Galen's Wax, 53
gel masks, 19
gels, 47
genderless branding, 117
Golden Rule, 9–10
Greeks, 52–53

H

hair removal, laser, 25–26
handwashing, 96
HEVL, 62
Hippocrates, 53
honey, 109
Huang Ti, 54
humectants, 44, 74
hyaluronic acid, 5, 21, 92
hypoallergenic, 80–81

I

inactive ingredients, 72–73
INCI. *See* International
  Nomenclature of Cosmetic
  Ingredients (INCI)
India, 53–54
intense pulsed light, 23–24

International Nomenclature of
  Cosmetic Ingredients (INCI),
  74
Isolaz, 24

J

jade roller, 41
Johnson's Baby Oil, 108
Juvéderm, 21

K

kids, 94–96

L

labels
  active ingredients in, 72–73
  ambiguous terms in, 80–82
  inactive ingredients in, 72–73
  ingredients with long names in,
    73–74
  order of ingredients in, 72
  symbols in, 79–80
laser hair removal, 25–26
laser therapy, 22–24
layering, in application, 9–10
Lemon Acne Spot Treatment, 113
light therapy, 41
lotions, 6, 46

M

makeup, 28, 91
makeup remover, 39
Maran, Josie, 54
masks, 17–20, 39, 102–103, 112

massage, 42
MEA, 77
melasma, 90
microdermabrasion, 14, 90
milk, 111
moisturizers, 6–8, 39, 43–47, 89, 92, 98–99, 112

N

natural, 82–84
niacinamide, 90
night creams, 34–38
nightly rituals, 31–42
Nivea Crème, 108
noncomedogenic, 80–81

O

oatmeal, steel-cut, 109
Oatmeal-Honey Gentle Skin Cleanser, 113
occlusives, 44–45
Oil of Olay, 108
oils, 7–8, 40, 50–55, 103–104
ointments, 46–47
Olay Moisturizing Lotion, 108
olive oil, 109
omega-3, 4–5
organic, 80, 83
oxybenzone, 78

P

parabens, 75–76
peel-off masks, 18–19
peptides, 4, 38, 75
Perlane, 21

Persia, 54
personalization, 116
petrolatum, 78
Photopneumatics, 24
phthalates, 76
Pliny the Elder, 52
Pond's Cold Cream, 106
potassium sorbate, 74
preservatives, as ingredient, 75
proteins, as ingredient, 75
puffiness, around eyes, 8

Q

Q-switched laser, 23

R

Radiesse, 21
Restylane, 21
retinol, 5, 38, 90
Romans, 52
rose, 114
rose quartz roller, 41

S

Sculptra, 21
sea salt, 110
serums, 4–5, 39, 91, 100–101
shortening, 110
showers, baths vs., 55–57
silicones, 77
SilkPeel, 22
sixties, 92–93
skin, 87
sleep, 32–34
soap

Notes

Notes